A Workbook for Trainees in General Practice

A Workbook for Trainees in General Practice

from the department of General Practice St George's Hospital Medical School

by Paul Freeling OBE MBBS FRCGP *Head of Department*

With the assistance of

Ralph Burton MBBS MRCGP	*Senior Tutor*
Richard Chegwidden AKC MBBS	*Senior Tutor*
Peter Fitton BSc MBBS MRCGP	*Research Fellow*
Clifford Floyd MBBS FRCGP	*Senior Tutor*
Lydia Smythe MBBS MRCGP	*Senior Tutor*

WRIGHT · PSG

Bristol London Boston

1983

Published by
John Wright & Sons Ltd, 823–825 Bath Road, Bristol
BS4 5NU, England

John Wright PSG Inc., 545 Great Road, Littleton,
Massachusetts 01460, U.S.A.

British Library Cataloguing in Publication Data

Freeling, Paul
A workbook for trainees in general practice.
1. Family medicine.
I. Title
362.1 '72 R729.5.G4

ISBN 0 7236 0681 1

Typeset and printed in Great Britain by
John Wright & Sons (Printing) Ltd
at The Stonebridge Press, Bristol BS4 5NU.

Preface

You have decided to train as a general practitioner. General practice has emerged as a discipline in its own right only recently. Like any other branch of medicine it has elements of science, craft and art in its make-up. You will find it easier to practise the science, produce work worthy of a craftsman and obtain the rewards of the art if you have a sound grounding in the basic skills of practice. This workbook is designed to outline some of these skills and help you make as effective a start to your training as possible. The book will be most helpful if you start using it immediately on joining your training practice. Whilst attached to the practice you will have a wide range of learning experiences, informal and formal. The more formal ones will include tutorials with your trainer, attendance at a release course and, perhaps, a trainer/trainee group. If you read the text, and undertake the sequence of tasks suggested, there should be three types of benefit:

1. You should find the transition from hospital practice to general practice less confusing than have some of your predecessors.

2. You and your trainer should be able to use efficiently and effectively selected tutorials in the early part of your training.

3. You should rapidly be able to join in discussions on the release course (and trainer/trainee group) where there will be doctors with more experience of general practice who have acquired already a language of ideas for expressing and meeting the educational needs they have identified.

The text also provides a useful, if incomplete, source of reference during the rest of your time in training.

You will have spent some time learning about general practice when you were a medical student and may find the approach taken towards the early tutorials rather simplistic. We would still suggest you work through them.

Two principles have been kept in mind when designing this workbook.

First, learning tends to be more effective when a 'need to know' has been recognized. If you examine the work you have to do you will uncover a need for information and approaches. Once you have gained extra knowledge you are more likely to retain it if you practise its use and are given feed-back about your success together with opportunities to extend it, correct it, or reject it.

The second principle is that if learning is to continue, not only in the period of your training, but throughout your professional life it is useful to have what are sometimes called 'models of the process of practice'. Examples in this workbook are the general problem-solving model (p. 58), and the preventive model (p. 103). All the models given in this workbook have been found useful by other GPs. How useful they are to you remains to be determined by your application of them to your work and learning from them. In general the value of models is that they are less likely to become outdated than are some of the facts to which they can be applied.

There will, nevertheless, be many facts which you will need to learn, even if they prove of transitory value. An extensive list of these will be found in *Learning and Teaching in General Practice*, a booklet prepared by the Scottish Council for Postgraduate Medical Education.

The range of topics which may be covered in your Release Course is outlined in Appendix C. It would be wise to obtain as soon as possible a programme for the Release Course which you will yourself attend.

In your tutorials you and your trainer may well derive models of your own which you can test out. These tutorials should last between 60 and 90 minutes. Themes to be dealt with should have been stipulated and both trainer and trainee should have prepared relevant material. Although the work of the practice will form an important part of the learning material for tutorials they are not meant to replace or be replaced by informal discussions which tend to arise *ad hoc* from that work.

It seems sensible to draw up a 'planner' for your time in the practice. Your plans are likely to be firmer earlier on and it is sensible to leave gaps with a frequency increasing with the time already spent there. This will allow for flexibility as you identify your 'need to know' from your experiences and with the help of your trainer.

The tutorials in this workbook are arranged so as to balance the apparently conflicting needs of a structure permitting preparation for them, and flexibility to allow for different experiences, different needs and different rates of learning.

Acknowledgements

Many people helped us and encouraged us to produce this workbook for GP trainees and we cannot mention them all by name. We must thank in particular Professor George Dick, lately Postgraduate Dean for South West Thames Region and his Adviser in General Practice, Dr Douglas Price, for arranging financial support which enabled us to test our ideas on a number of trainers and trainees. Without their help our task would have been most difficult.

Mrs Sheila Skipp and Miss Sue Nash have patiently, and with remarkable accuracy, typed version after version. We owe them a great deal.

Our families have tolerated our obsession: we are grateful.

We have been much helped by our medical students whose observations and contribution to discussion helped form our thoughts.

Contents

How to use the workbook

Scan through the workbook and see if you think its approach is logical. If you have any difficulties raise them with your Trainer at the beginning of Tutorial I or with your Course Organizer at your first attendance at the release course.

After you have scanned the workbook read carefully that part which concerns Tutorial I, study the tasks and any forms relating to them. The forms are presented in miniature but you can draw them up in a larger format for your own use. Ask your trainer about the tasks if there is anything you do not understand. Complete the form(s); repeat your reading of the text and share Tutorial I. Repeat this sequence for each tutorial.

It will be best if the forms only are taken into the surgery so that you can make notes without it being too obvious to the patient. You may decide that some of the forms are best completed after the surgery has ended using notes you have made during the consultations. The forms are intended to help you focus on and bring material relevant to the next tutorial.

Do not hesitate to ask your trainer, *ad hoc*, any clinical questions which arise during shared surgery sessions or visits.

You should look carefully at the appendices, especially Appendix A which describes the essentials of a contract for trainees.

Part A

Settling into Practice

Tutorial I What is general practice?

In this first section we look at general practice within its context, summarize the aims of your training and take a first look at workload in terms of numbers and diversity. Having read the text complete Form A before your first tutorial.

General practice is a term used for a number of purposes; as a consequence there is often confusion when general practice is discussed.

A. JOB DESCRIPTION

An operational definition of general practice is that it is the special set of knowledge, skills and attitudes which should be possessed if the job description of the general practitioner is to be met. The Councils for Postgraduate Medical Education have selected as the job description to which your training will be directed one which is widely accepted in Europe. It reads:

> 'The general practitioner is a licensed medical graduate who gives care to individuals, irrespective of age, sex and illness. He will attend his patients in his consulting room and in their homes and sometimes in a clinic or a hospital. His aim is to make early diagnoses. He will include and integrate physical, psychological, and social factors in his considerations about health and illness. He will make an initial decision about every problem which is presented to him as a doctor. He will undertake the continuing management of his patients with chronic, recurrent or terminal illnesses. Prolonged contact means that he can use repeated opportunities to gather information at a pace appropriate to each patient and build up a relationship of trust which he can use professionally. He will practise in co-operation with other colleagues, medical and non-medical. He will know how and when to intervene through treatment, prevention and education to promote the health of his patients and their families. He will recognize that he also has a professional

responsibility to the community.' *Leeuwenhorst Working Party* (1974).

B. POSITION IN A BUREAUCRACY

A second operational definition of general practice is that it forms part of the primary tier of medical care which is provided in Great Britain within a two-tier system. Community physicians and clinical medical officers also work in the primary tier. The two-tier system is now formalized in the National Health Service where most medical care in Great Britain is obtained. The secondary tier is provided by doctors working in or from hospital, usually within a specialty. They usually see only patients who are referred to them by primary-tier doctors.

The activities of general practice care include:

First-contact care
Continuing care
Preventive care

C. A PLACE IN A COMMUNITY

A third operational definition of general practice is that it comprises a building, the staff who work in and from it, and the defined list of patients for whom they provide care. The defined list is an important consequence of the NHS. Another important consequence is that the care is obtained 'free-at-the-time'. Both consequences offer a GP in the NHS unusual opportunities to conduct preventive and continuing aspects of care as well as removing financial obstacles to the patient making first-contact with the practice. A further consequence of the formal two-tier system now embodied in the NHS is that higher technologies, which can form an essential part of medical care, tend to be restricted to hospitals to which patients who use them must be referred. 'Open access' is, however, provided by hospitals for GPs to many of the techniques used for investigating patients. 'Open access' means that GPs can request an investigation without the intervention of a hospital clinician. The boundaries between general practice and hospitals change constantly as technology advances. A simple example is that many GPs now possess their own electrocardiograms whilst some hospital ECG services have yet to be made 'open access'.

D. SPECIAL INTERESTS

Many GPs extend their involvement in medicine outside the job definition. GPs often fill part-time jobs providing medical services in the community but outside general practice. The responsibilities of these posts can vary widely; not all are concerned with providing care. Some GPs work in part-time posts in hospital, others have hospital beds in their own charge. Many GPs undertake voluntary work. Those GPs who undertake it feel that this outside work adds to their job satisfaction. In some partnerships individual GPs emphasize a narrower component of their work (such as contraceptive advice or assessment of child development) but, usually, not to the complete exclusion of that part of their job definition which states that he or she will 'make an initial decision about every problem which is presented to him as a doctor'. Unless the attitudes described in the educational aims of your training are demonstrated by the doctor when following a special interest the work done should not be called a part of general practice. Special interests within the practice are followed within the framework of general practice in its various operational definitions. This framework results in a number of characteristics, the *combination* of which throughout the developed world makes general practice the unique discipline it is.

Compared to hospital medicine general practice is a low technology discipline, taking a person-orientated rather than a disease-orientated approach to medical care. As patients have direct contact with the doctor its practitioners deal with undifferentiated illness and may be responsible for helping the patient organize their symptoms. The care of the patient continues after the episode of illness which makes prevention an important part of primary care. Continuing care needs a knowledge of development and of the natural history of disease. One of its principal diagnostic and therapeutic tools is the use of time, which, if it is to be used properly, requires an understanding of the probabilities and threats in decision making, and the ability to tolerate uncertainty.

The principal work area of general practice is the consultation which calls for high skills in interviewing. The doctor requires knowledge of other professionals, both within his own practice team and outside, and to use their skills selectively. Whilst the primary duty is to the patient the doctor's responsibility to the whole community cannot be ignored.

Practice within the NHS means that the GP acts in the above way for a defined 'list' of patients. In providing their care he has control of large sums of money by prescribing and certification and also exerts control over scarce hospital resources by his referral rate.

Because doctors and patients remain individuals there are problems with the maintenance of standards and the acceptance of advice.

These *Characteristics of General Practice* are:

1. Undifferentiated illness.
2. Patients helped to 'organize' their illnesses (Balint, 1957).
3. Low technology.
4. Use of estimates of probabilities and threats (Royal College of General Practitioners, 1977).
5. Use of 'time'.
6. Person-centred approach (Tait, 1974).
7. Problems of compliance both for doctors and patients.
8. Continuing care.
9. Preventive attitude.
10. Developmental approach.
11. Selective use of resources.
12. Responsibility to whole community.
13. Need to tolerate uncertainty (Thomson, 1978).
14. Knowledge of other disciplines.
15. High skills in interviewing.
16. Care of defined 'list'
17. Control over money and resources

} NHS characteristics.

Responsive and responsible

The characteristics listed mean that general practice is both responsible and responsive. The responsive nature of the work means that the flow of work varies to an extent with the characteristics of the community served, and that organization of the work varies also, partly because of community characteristics, partly because GPs themselves vary. Although a GP may work in the same building as other doctors in a health centre or in group practice premises, and may have partners, by habit he works very much alone. Only relatively recently has the concept of a Primary Health Care Team begun to spread through the profession, and the increase in the number of vocational trainees is even more recent. Hospital doctors have long been accountable to each other for their decisions and actions; few GPs have much practice, yet, in responding to requests to justify their work and methods. Your trainer, and by association any partners, have agreed to do this by taking on the responsibility of helping you to manage your learning.

EDUCATIONAL AIMS OF YOUR TRAINING

The educational aims of your training, the set of knowledge, skills and attitudes you should have acquired, require you to be able to demonstrate at the end of your training that:

1. Knowledge

a. You have sufficient knowledge of disease processes, particularly of common diseases, chronic diseases and those which endanger life or have serious complications or consequences.
b. You understand the opportunities, methods and limitations of prevention, early diagnosis and management in the setting of general practice.
c. You understand the way in which interpersonal relationships within the family can cause health problems or alter their presentation, course and management, just as illness can influence family relationships.
d. You understand the social and environmental circumstances of your patients and how they may affect health and illness.
e. You know and can use appropriately the wide range of interventions available to you.
f. You understand the ethics of your profession and their importance for the patient.
g. You understand the basic methods of research as applied to general practice.
h. You understand medico-social legislation and the impact of this on your patient.

2. Skills

a. You can form diagnoses which take account of physical, psychological and social factors.
b. You understand the use of epidemiology and probability in your everyday work.

c. You understand and can use the factor 'time' as a diagnostic, therapeutic and organizational tool.
d. You can identify persons at risk and take appropriate action.
e. You can make relevant initial decisions about every problem presented to you as a doctor.
f. You can co-operate with medical and non-medical professionals.
g. You know and make appropriate use of the skills of practice management.

3. Attitudes

a. You possess a capacity for empathy and for forming a specific and effective relationship with patients and for developing a degree of self-understanding.
b. Your recognition of the patient as a unique individual modifies the ways in which you elicit information and make hypotheses about the nature of problems and their management.
c. You understand that helping patients to solve their own problems is a fundamental therapeutic activity.
d. You recognize that you can make a professional contribution to the wider community.
e. You are willing and able to evaluate your own work critically.
f. You recognize your own need for continuing education and critical reading of medical information.

CATEGORIZING CONSULTATIONS

David Morrell, Wolfson Professor of General Practice at St Thomas' Hospital Medical School, has suggested two simple ways of categorizing consultations. The first way is by the arrangements which precede the patient/doctor contact; the second way is by the doctor's judgement of the severity of the condition (Morrell et al., 1971).

1. Arrangements made for consultation

'*New*' consultations, initiated by the patient for an episode not previously the subject of a consultation, have been estimated to make up 25 per cent of an established principal's work in a well-organized practice.

'*Repeat*' consultations, initiated by the GP for short-term follow-up of an acute condition, long-term follow-up for a chronic condition, or preventive activities, have been estimated to make up 50 per cent of the work of the same sort of GP. These consultations are entirely within the control of the GP.

'*Recidivist*' consultations, initiated by the patient but concerning a matter which the GP considered finished with, make up the remaining 25 per cent of the work.

The term 'recidivist' has unpleasant connotations since *The Concise Oxford Dictionary* defines it as 'one who relapses into crime'. Perhaps you would like to consider why such an emotive word was chosen to describe this group. If you think it is inappropriate, coin a phrase of your own.

2. How severe are the conditions seen?

A '*minor*' condition is defined as one which is self-limiting and carries no threat to life nor risk of permanent disability; 65 per cent of clinical diagnoses made by GPs seem to concern minor conditions.

A '*major*' condition is defined as one carrying a reasonable chance of threatening life or risk of being followed by permanent disability; 15 per cent of the clinical diagnoses made by GPs concern such major conditions.

A '*chronic*' condition is one which carries a threat of downhill progress or a state of reduced function; 20 per cent of GPs' clinical work deals with chronic conditions.

We suggest that you complete Form A before Tutorial I. Doing so will help you to examine some of the ideas discussed in the text.

The form enables you to record three items about each patient attending the surgery: first, how was the consultation arranged? second, was the condition acute or chronic? and third, if acute, was the condition minor or major?

You should record one morning and one evening surgery spent with your trainer.

Tutorial I Form A

Name Code	M/F	Age	Arrangements			Reason			
						Acute			
			New	Rpt	Recd	Minor	Major	Chronic	Detail

LABELLING

You will have found it possible to label firmly many of the consultations you have witnessed within the categories suggested. You may have had some difficulty in deciding what was 'major' and what was 'minor'. Any difficulty may have resulted from differences between your perception of the problem presented and the perception of the patient. In addition, you will have noticed that few consultations have a content all of which can be labelled in terms of the disease labels used in the data lists as representing minor, major and chronic illness. The unlabelled content usually reflects psychological and social factors. This workbook offers opportunities during later tutorials for discussion of all these difficulties in categorization.

After you have completed Form A for a morning and an evening surgery you should contrast your findings with the following data which has been calculated for a practice population of 2500 people. It is taken from *Trends in General Practice, 1979* (*see* Appendix, G, Basic Reading List) although the data was first published in 1975.

Age/sex structure of average practice

	Male (%)	*Female* (%)	*Total* (%)
0– 4 years (Pre-school child)	8·4	7·6	8·0
5–15 years (School child)	16·5	14·9	16·7
16–45 years (Young adult)	40·2	37·1	38·6
46–64 years (Middle-aged adult)	24·1	24·4	24·2
65+ years (Elderly)	10·5	16·0	13·2
All ages	48·6	51·4	

In a year the following events would be likely to occur in a population of 2500.

Births	32
Marriages	17
Divorces	5
Deaths	25

Social pathology in a practice of 2500

Conditions		*Persons*
Aged		
Over 65 (at risk)		375
Over 75 (at risk)		100
'Poor' receiving supplementary social benefit		150
Severe physical handicaps		70
Deaf	25	
Blind	10	
Severe mental handicaps		60
Schizophrenics	5	
Alcoholics	10	
One-parent families		27
Unemployed		31
Problem families		10
Juvenile delinquents		7
Divorce		5
Illegitimate births		3
Adults in prison		4

Major illness in a practice of 2500

Conditions		*Persons consulting per year*
Acute bronchitis		100
Pneumonia		20
Severe depression		10
Suicide attempt	3	
Suicide	1 every 4 years	
Acute myocardial infarction		8
Acute appendicitis		5
Acute strokes		5
ALL new cancers		5
Lung	2 per year	
Breast	1 per year	
Large bowel	2 every 3 years	
Stomach	1 every 2 years	
Prostate	1 every 2 years	
Bladder	1 every 3 years	
Cervix	1 every 4 years	
Ovary	1 every 5 years	
Oesophagus	1 every 7 years	
Brain	1 every 10 years	
Uterine body	1 every 12 years	
Lymphadenoma	1 every 15 years	
Thyroid	1 every 20 years	

Minor illness in a practice of 2500

Conditions	*Persons consulting per year*
General	
Upper respiratory infections	600
Skin disorders	325
Emotional disorders	300
Gastro-intestinal disorders	200
Specific	
Acute tonsillitis	100
Acute otitis media	75
Cerumen	50
Acute urinary infections	50
'Acute back' syndrome	50
Migraine	25
Hay fever	25

Chronic disease in a practice of 2500

Conditions		*Persons consulting per year*
Chronic rheumatism		100
Rheumatoid arthritis	10	
Osteoarthritis of hips	5	
Chronic mental illness		60
High blood pressure		50
Obesity		40
Chronic bronchitis		35
Anaemia		
Iron deficiency		25
Pernicious anaemia		4
Chronic heart failure		30
Cancers		30
Asthma		25
Peptic ulcers		20
Coronary artery disease		20
Cerebrovascular disease		15
Epilepsy		10
Diabetes		10
Thyroid disease		7
Parkinsonism		3
Multiple sclerosis		2
Chronic renal failure		less than 1

Congenital disorders expected in a population of 2500

Conditions	*Expected in a population of 2500*	
Heart lesion	1 new case every	5 years
Pyloric stenosis	1 new case every	7 years
Spina bifida	1 new case every	7 years
Mongolism	1 new case every	10 years
Cleft palate	1 new case every	20 years
Dislocated hip	1 new case every	10 years
Phenylketonuria	1 new case every	200 years

You should now be prepared for Tutorial I with your trainer with the theme 'What is general practice?'.

During the tutorial you should be able to make an initial exploration of the ways in which your time in the training practice can help you to achieve the aims of your training for general practice.

You should refer also to individual consultations which illustrate some of the points made in the text.

Tutorial II How do the internal arrangements of the practice and its setting affect the work done?

In this section we are concerned with the running of the practice (arrangements), with its premises and its geographical location (setting). Setting and arrangements tend, of course, to interact with each other and with the work done.

Forms B1 and B2 and the practice map should bring these details into focus for your practice.

You have looked at the work of general practice in two ways: how patients arranged to see the doctor; and whether the problem which patients brought to the doctor was acute or chronic, major or minor. It is self-evident that the arrangements made by patients will depend upon the way in which the practice is organized and staffed (**structure**). The structure of a practice is likely to affect the nature of the conditions which patients bring to their GPs as is the nature of the population served (**demography**) and the housing and transport systems available to the population (**setting**). The three factors, structure, demography and setting, reflect the operational definitions of general practice already given.

A. WHAT IS THE STRUCTURE OF THE PRACTICE?

The term 'structure' is taken from a proposal by Donabedian (1977) that the study of medical care services can be of three areas, structure, process and outcome. The matter of medical audit in general practice, and some illustrative examples, will be touched upon in later tutorials. What must be stated now is that, in general practice 'structure' usually refers to such elements as the doctor–patient ratio, the membership of the primary care team, the provision of diagnostic facilities and of special clinics, and the premises available.

The internal arrangements of practices vary considerably. The variation stems from the bureaucratic arrangements made for the provision of general medical services within the NHS. The general practitioner has the status of an individual entrepreneur within the NHS in contrast to the status of hospital doctors who, whatever their level of responsibility, are salaried employees. This difference in status will have important financial consequences for you when you eventually become a principal: it will affect both the amount of money you will have for personal use and the way in which it is taxed. Knowledge of financial matters and an understanding of accounting and tax procedures are essential to your achieving by the end of your training for general practice Aim 2(*g*) (*see* p. 10), concerning knowledge and appropriate use of the skills of practice management. It is inappropriate to focus on details of payment and reimbursement at this stage of your training: you will find useful information in Appendix B. Other, more detailed texts for reference are: *The Red Book*: the Statement of Fees and Allowances provided to all GPs by the Family Practitioner Committee with whom they are in contract; the *Blue Book* produced by 'Pulse', and a book from the Department of General Practice at Exeter University entitled *Running A Practice*, Jones R. V. H., Bolden K. J., Gray D. J. P. and Hall M. S. (1978) London, Croom Helm.

1. The doctor–patient ratio

The average list size of GPs in England on 1 October 1976 was 2351. The average in the South-West of England was 2181, as compared with the East Midlands where it was 2460.

GPs may practice in groups or be single-handed. There has been a strong trend in the UK for doctors to work in groups and for these groups to become larger. In October 1976 the 20 551 GPs in England worked in 8924 general practices.

The distribution of practices of differing size is shown below:

Group size	1	2	3	4	5+
1976	39%	23%	19%	11%	8%

Put another way the following are the percentages of GPs in various size groups:

Group size	1	2	3	4	5+
1976	17%	20%	24%	18%	21%

There is a general tendency for there to be more single-handed practices the nearer a locality is to the centre of large cities. In 1977, 27 per cent of practices in London were single-handed compared to the national average of 16 per cent. There are four London Family Practitioner Committees which are truly 'inner city': Camden and Islington, and City and East London, both with 35 per cent of GPs single-handed; Kensington, Chelsea and Westminster, where 56 per cent were; and Lambeth, Southwark and Lewisham, where 32 per cent of GPs were single-handed (Royal College of General Practitioners, 1981).

It is obvious that the tendency described for single-handed practices to be found with increased frequencies near the centres of large cities does not result generally from a paucity of patients although it may do so in such localities as the City of London where there is very little domestic accommodation. The tendency reflects, therefore, other aspects, three of which are opportunities for work outside general practice, individual idiosyncracies of the doctors concerned and the availability of practice premises.

2. Premises and staff

In the past GPs usually owned their own practice premises—often living in them—or on occasions rented from a private landlord. More recently health centres have been built by local authorities to house their own staff as well as providing accommodation for local GPs. A health centre may have practising from it a group of GPs, partnerships, or single-handed doctors. The need for larger premises than can normally be provided from a house in which the doctor and his family also lives reflects the move towards the use of ancillary and nursing staff and the primary care team, as well as the expectations of both doctor and patient for the provision of a wider range of care than formerly. In particular, it reflects the extension of general practice from an acute episodic service, albeit within a framework of continuity of care, into preventive and anticipatory care as well as the care of chronic disability.

The increase in the range of tasks undertaken in general practice is one of the reasons why many GPs have set up appointment systems, run clinics outside normal consulting hours, and delegate to other members of the primary health care team as well as accepting delegation from them.

Nursing help

The notion of using the skills of nurses to extend the capability of general practice is of long standing. When local authorities began, in the 19th century, to employ qualified nurses to work in the homes of patients in a specified district they probably did so to supplement services provided by doctors but not in an integrated manner. The responsibility for continuing to provide a district nursing service was laid upon local authorities in the original National Health Service Acts. The Health Service and Public Health Act of 1968 encouraged district nurses to attend patients also in general practitioners' surgeries and in clinics. This enactment recognized the tendency which had developed for GPs and district nurses to work together and develop the concept of the primary care team on which Tutorial III will concentrate. The 1968 National Health Service Act led to an increase in the 'attachment' of District Nurses to general practice. By 1978, 67 per cent of practices had nurses attached.

There have always been some GPs who themselves employed nurses to work in their surgeries. The number of practices doing so increased after the NHS arranged, in 1966, to partially reimburse the salaries of staff employed by GPs.

By 1975, 24 per cent of general practices in England employed one or more nurses: by 1980, 27 per cent did so.

The trend towards attachment of District Nurses to general practices has recently been attacked, and in some areas reversed. The trend towards the directly employed practice nurse has also been attacked. The range of work of both kinds of nurses has recently been studied (Reedy et al., 1980a,b). Reedy and his colleagues divide the possible clinical activities of nurses working with GPs into three categories: *caring*, such as bathing patients and administering medicines; *technical*, such as syringing ears, performing ECGs and skin testing for allergies; and *intermediate*, such as removing sutures and giving counsel and support. The frequency of these activities and their distribution between the two types of nurses, health authority employed and practice employed, will be discussed in the text relevant to Tutorial III. What must be emphasized in this section which is preparatory for Tutorial II is that the range of activities undertaken is related to the physical structure of the practice premises.

Accommodation

In 1969, 71 per cent of GPs in health centres and 31 per cent of those in other premises had a treatment room. By 1977, 96 per cent of GPs in health centres and 77 per cent of others had a treatment room.

It is clear that there are many other ways in which the physical structure of the practice affects the work done by the staff employed. This applies to the doctors as much as to other members of the primary care team and includes equipment as well as the availability of space.

Staff employed

a. You will realize that, like most other doctors, the GP works in association with other people, some of whom are trained in caring professions, some of whom have a background of secretarial skills.
b. The GP is reimbursed 70 per cent of the salaries of those staff he/she employs.
c. The DHA and Local Authority employed staff may be attached to the practice (i.e. have responsibility only for the GP's patients) or have geographical responsibility (i.e. be associated with a number of different practices).

Detailed descriptions of the work of the District Nurse, Health Visitor and Social Worker will be found in the text for Tutorial III. The work of GP employees such as a practice nurse and of secretarial staff varies from practice to practice.

3. Diagnostic Equipment

Since 1970 there has been a huge increase in the availability of ready-sterilized and disposable diagnostic items, such as vaginal specula which has been paralleled by miniaturization and other technological advances which have made it possible for GPs to perform in their surgeries more detailed investigation of their patients. You will now know the range of equipment available in your training practice. It would be interesting to compare it with that reported as being in the possession of teachers in 1981. In the following table are given also the percentage of teachers in 1970 and in 1969 of a random sample of GPs reporting the same equipment. (In 1970 organized vocational training for general practice was innovatory and experimental: since then it has become accepted and now mandatory.)

Equipment

	Percentage Possessing		
		Teaching practices	
Item	All practices 1969*	1970*	1981†
Vaginal speculum	68	97	100
Proctoscope	70	94	94
Refrigerator	69	87	99
Sterilizer	—	86	97
For minor surgery	78	83	89
Arm balance weighing machine	—	52	79
Baby scales	—	49	87
Microscope	34	49	64
Haemoglobinometer	35	37	30
Laryngoscope	26	37	46
ECG	10	37	69
Peak flow meter	5	28	87
Cautery apparatus	—	27	50
Audiometer	—	12	35
Sigmoidoscope	—	12	18
Centrifuge	—	11	13

* 1969 and 1970 data from Irvine D. H. Teaching practices. Report from General Practice 15. *Journal of the Royal College of General Practitioners*, June 1972.
† 1981 data unpublished.

4. Arrangements

The varying arrangements made by practices reflect the staff and premises available. With increasing frequency, patients are seen by appointment (6 per cent of all practices in 1961, 30 per cent in 1967 and 64 per cent in 1972). Some patients feel that GPs use appointment systems as hurdles rather than as gates; that it has become more difficult rather than easier to see a doctor since these systems were introduced. Some GPs feel that appointment systems put them under pressure to work faster than they like.

The introduction of group practice and of appointment systems, like the undertaking of work outside general practice, reflects the statutory responsibilities placed upon GPs by their contracts with the NHS. They contract to have a personal responsibility 24 hours a day, 365 days a year to each patient registered with them and undertake to provide care, at least at first contact, for all conditions which the *patient* identifies as medical. This contractual responsibility reflects the responsibilities stated more clearly in the job definition.

As the job definition indicates, the basic work area of general practice, the consultation, may take place in the consulting room, in the patient's home or even in hospital. The number of consultations is normally expressed as consultation/1000 patients registered/year. Figures vary widely from 3000/1000 to 4500/1000. The 'average GP' then has 7500 consultations with patients per year. There is surprisingly little variation, however, in reports of length of consultation: whilst an average duration of 5 minutes is often stated, an average of 6–7 minutes is usually reported in surveys of surgery consultation. Consultations in the home are felt by many GPs to be an essential part of general practice in the UK—these doctors feel that they obtain essential information about their patients and their families on such visits. Nevertheless, the percentage of consultations conducted in the home has fallen steadily over the years, although there is great variation in totals from practice to practice. Few GPs would expect to have more than 4–6 home consultations a day unless an epidemic was raging.

One of the most onerous of the GP's responsibilities is that of providing care 'out-of-hours'. There is special payment made by the NHS to GPs for each visit to a patient at home made between 11.00 p.m. and 7.00 a.m. The total of such claims gives an average of 10 such calls per GP per year, although it is realized that there is underclaiming. Many different arrangements are made for 'out-of-hours' calls ranging from a single-handed doctor always 'on call' through in-practice rotas and inter-practice rotas to the employment of organized commercial call services.

We suggest that you record the staffing structure of your training practice on Form B1. You should interview each member of staff and determine what they see as their tasks within the practice.

Form B1. **Practice Profile**

Is the practice

a. Single-handed?
b. Group practice?
c. Health Centre practice?

If *b* and *c*:

Number of doctors in practice

a. Principals ____________________
b. Assistants ____________________
c. Trainees ____________________

Members of staff (please give numbers) Names (underline how usually addressed)

1. *Other caring professions*
   - Practice nurse ____________________
   - District nurse ____________________
   - Health visitor ____________________
   - Midwife ____________________
   - Social worker ____________________
   - Physiotherapist ____________________
   - Chiropodist ____________________
   - Dietitian ____________________
2. *Secretarial Staff*
   - Practice manager ____________________
   - Book-keeper ____________________
   - Receptionist ____________________
   - Typist ____________________
   - Filing clerk ____________________

You should, at the same time, record the physical structure of your training practice on Form B2.

Form B2. **Practice 'Structure'**

PREMISES

Is there: Tick if yes

1. An examination room attached to each consulting room?
2. A treatment room other than consulting or exam room?
3. Health visitors room?
4. Separate records room?
5. Separate secretary or office manager's room?
6. Number of consulting rooms?
7. Other rooms?

Appointment system: YES/NO FULL/PARTIAL (please ring)
If 'YES'

a. Frequency of appointments No. ________/________min

b. Please describe the arrangements for patients without appointments who need to be seen the same day.

c. Describe the arrangements made for home visiting by the GPs.

B. WHAT IS THE DEMOGRAPHY OF THE PRACTICE?

The demographical characteristics of a practice which are likely to affect its work-load and the nature of the care it provides include: The doctor–patient ratio; the proportions of its defined list which fall into different age/sex categories; and the distribution of its population in terms of social class.

Some data concerning doctor–patient ratios have been given already.

1. Age and sex

Your practice may have an age/sex register. This will permit you to describe in these terms the patients for whom the practice is responsible. If there is no age/sex register you can determine the proportion of patients between 65 and 74 and the proportion who are 75 and over from the payment sheets issued to your trainer (and his partner(s)) each quarter. Extra payment is made to GPs in regard of these two categories of patient which suggests that they are expected

Patients consulting, showing frequency of consultation by sex and age for persons at risk for the whole study year. All practices

Frequency of consultation	All ages (%)	0–4 (%)	5–14 (%)	15–24 (%)	25–44 (%)	45–64 (%)	65–74 (%)	75+ (%)
				Males				
Nil	39·8	20·4	37·8	43·4	44·1	41·1	37·7	35·6
1	17·2	16·8	21·2	19·7	17·5	14·1	13·4	13·8
2	11·7	13·9	13·9	12·3	11·4	10·2	9·9	8·5
3	8·0	12·1	9·0	7·7	7·6	7·1	7·4	8·0
4	5·7	8·7	5·8	5·4	5·0	5·8	5·8	5·0
5	4·1	6·9	3·8	3·5	3·6	4·2	4·6	4·1
6	2·9	5·3	2·7	2·2	2·4	3·1	3·5	3·8
7	2·3	3·9	1·8	1·6	1·9	2·7	3·0	3·3
8	1·7	3·0	1·1	1·2	1·4	1·9	2·3	2·6
9	1·2	2·2	0·7	0·8	1·0	1·6	1·9	2·3
10–14	3·3	5·0	1·7	1·5	2·7	4·7	5·9	6·5
15–19	1·2	1·3	0·3	0·4	0·9	1·9	2·4	3·4
20–29	0·6	0·4	0·1	0·1	0·5	1·1	1·5	1·9
30–49	0·1	0·0	0·0	0·0	0·1	0·3	0·4	0·8
50 and over	0·0	0·0	0·0	0·0	0·0	0·1	0·1	0·3
Total persons registered (= 100%)	129 397	8892	23 322	18 970	33 554	31 795	8784	3980
				Females				
Nil	32·4	22·1	36·7	28·9	29·8	34·7	36·3	34·9
1	15·1	16·9	21·3	14·7	13·3	14·4	12·5	12·0
2	11·7	15·5	14·1	11·5	11·3	11·0	9·8	9·4
3	8·7	11·5	9·4	8·9	9·0	8·2	7·4	6·7
4	6·7	8·5	6·0	7·3	6·9	6·4	6·2	5·5
5	5·1	6·6	3·9	5·4	5·7	4·9	4·7	4·6
6	3·8	4·5	2·6	4·2	4·4	3·7	3·8	3·7
7	3·1	3·8	1·9	3·4	3·4	3·2	3·0	3·5
8	2·5	2·8	1·2	2·8	2·9	2·5	2·5	2·7
9	2·0	2·2	0·8	2·2	2·3	2·1	2·2	2·7
10–14	5·5	4·2	1·7	6·5	6·7	5·6	6·8	7·8
15–19	2·0	0·9	0·3	2·7	2·6	1·9	2·6	3·3
20–29	1·1	0·3	1·1	1·3	1·4	1·0	1·5	2·3
30–49	0·3	0·0	—	0·2	0·2	0·3	0·6	0·8
50 and over	0·0	—	—	0·0	0·0	0·1	0·1	0·2
Total persons registered (= 100%)	140 435	8493	21 981	19 097	35 757	33 985	12 428	8694

to make more demands upon general medical services than some other age groups.

The Second National Morbidity Study from general practice showed a number of interesting contrasts. About one-third of patients had no consultation in the study year. Women aged 15–44 were much more likely to consult than men of the same age. Frequent attendance (seven or more consultations a year) was twice as common among women as among men aged 15–44. The adjoining table gives the full data.

2. Social class

Patients can be allocated to social class in a number of ways. A very specific way is for purposes of epidemiology—the Registrar-General's Classification. This depends upon occupation, and in the case of married women it is their husband's occupation which defines class. Other systems, often more easily applicable in everyday clinical practice, derive from judgements of the norms and values which people manifest as characteristics of the culture of the social class to which they belong. We recommend you to read during your trainee year *An Introduction to Medical Sociology* edited by David Tuckett and we make no attempt to summarize its contents here. The importance of social class as an apparent determinant of health and the effect the social class make-up of a practice may have on its work-flow is indicated by the next set of tables the first three of which concern mortality.

Standardized mortality ratios of men, married women (by husband's occupation), and single women, aged 15–64, by social class

	Social class (R.G.60)					
Group	I	II	III	IV	V	All
Men, 15–64 years	76	81	100	103	143	100
Women, married, 15–64 years	77	83	103	105	141	100
Women, single, 15–64 years	83	88	90	108	121	100

(*Derived from Table 1*, Decennial Supplement, England and Wales, 1961, 1971).

Mean annual death rate per 100 000 men by age group and social class

	Social class (R.G.60)					
Age group	I	II	III	IV	V	All men
15–19	67	99	90	110	132	93
20–24	67	97	103	114	170	114
25–34	82	81	100	119	202	112
35–44	166	177	234	251	436	241
45–54	535	545	708	734	1119	707
55–64	1699	1820	2218	2202	2912	2171
65–74	4666	5100	6347	5702	6715	5452

(*Derived from Table 3A(i)*, Decennial Supplement, England and Wales, 1961, 1971).

Comparison of social class standardized mortality ratios SMRs for selected causes, in men and married women aged 15–64

	Social class (R.G.60)									
	Men's social class					Women's social class				
Cause	I	II	III	IV	V	I	II	III	IV	V
Tuberculosis	40	54	96	108	185	41	61	102	112	178
Diabetes	81	103	100	98	122	43	67	95	121	183
Coronary disease	98	95	106	96	112	69	81	103	107	143
Influenza	58	67	89	114	162	46	74	97	121	171
Pneumonia	48	54	88	102	196	64	69	95	114	172
Bronchitis	28	50	97	116	194	33	51	102	118	196
Pneumoconiosis (occupational)	5	9	109	181	95	—	—	—	—	—
Appendicitis	104	79	104	105	108	80	98	104	100	108
Cirrhosis of liver	106	136	86	85	137	94	132	92	92	115
Accidents in home	95	78	81	104	226	107	91	87	99	171

N.B. SMRs refer to males and females separately; in each case the SMR for all social classes is 100; social class of married women is based on husband's occupation.
(*Derived from Table E1*, Decennial Supplement, England and Wales, 1961, 1971).

The differences in morbidity are even greater than those in mortality and some aspects are instanced in the following table.

Long-standing illness (limiting long-standing illness in brackets) (rates per 1000) CS 1971–76

	1970[a]	1972[b]	1973	1974	1975	1976
Males						
Professional	(90)	153 (72)	133 (57)	141 (82)	168 (93)	176 (80)
Employers and managers	(165)	173 (94)	187 (92)	185 (113)	216 (131)	215 (121)
Intermediate	(187)	185 (101)	224 (122)	226 (147)	229 (150)	245 (149)
Skilled manual	(188)	198 (114)	195 (109)	202 (132)	227 (143)	249 (160)
Semi-skilled manual	(245)	241 (146)	217 (133)	222 (147)	268 (162)	276 (178)
Unskilled manual	(334)	300 (209)	283 (190)	308 (225)	331 (227)	345 (234)
	(109)	197 (115)	201 (113)	206 (134)	231 (144)	245 (153)
Females						
Professional	(114)	104 (58)	117 (61)	154 (93)	149 (76)	177 (86)
Employers and managers	(155)	163 (86)	162 (82)	176 (115)	212 (124)	206 (131)
Intermediate	(157)	198 (106)	212 (119)	222 (143)	244 (152)	266 (163)
Skilled manual	(192)	185(111)	180 (103)	198 (124)	216 (139)	228 (143)
Semi-skilled manual	(279)	285 (176)	250 (157)	280 (198)	293 (197)	312 (213)
Unskilled manual	(340)	333 (206)	323 (203)	314 (229)	377 (263)	435 (299)
	(206)	215 (215)	210 (123)	224 (150)	246 (159)	264 (170)

[a] England and Wales, those aged 15 or over only, limiting long-standing illness only.
[b] England and Wales.
From Reports of the General Household Survey summarized in *Inequalities in Health*, 1981.

Although the rates given come from outdated surveys the relationship between them are likely to persist despite increasing affluence. This is because life-styles which result from class differences are resistant to change.

GP (NHS) consultations* by sex and socio-economic group, 1971–76

All persons	1971†	1972†	1973	1974	1975	1976
a. Persons consulting: rates per 1000						
Males						
Professional	86	87	84	82	85	96
Employers and managers	100	96	82	85	83	89
Intermediate and junior non-manual	93	91	97	96	96	92
Skilled manual (incl. foremen and supervisors) and own account non-professional	97	95	100	100	95	94
Semi-skilled and manual and personal service	105	115	102	120	104	87
Unskilled manual	110	137	122	116	94	107
Females						
Professional	—	119	90	120	114	110
Employers and managers	—	109	105	118	119	111
Intermediate and junior non-manual	—	134	123	124	126	131
Skilled manual (incl. foremen and supervisors) and own account non-professional	—	133	117	129	115	113
Semi-skilled manual and personal service	—	134	132	132	135	128
Unskilled manual	—	133	127	148	126	127
b. Consultations: rates per 1000						
Males						
Professional	100	110	100	101	104	114
Employers and managers	124	123	107	104	103	118
Intermediate and junior non-manual	115	113	121	116	119	112
Skilled manual (incl. foremen and supervisors) and own account non-professional	122	126	132	126	117	118
Semi-skilled manual and personal service	133	145	125	147	134	104
Unskilled manual	143	193	164	148	126	142
Females						
Professional	—	151	107	145	136	131
Employers and managers	—	141	128	149	136	130
Intermediate and junior non-manual	—	166	150	148	160	152
Skilled manual (incl. foremen and supervisors) and own account non-professional	—	170	140	149	137	139
Semi-skilled manual and personal service	—	163	161	160	167	149
Unskilled manual	—	177	161	174	145	133

* Consultations in a 2-week reference period. † England and Wales only.
From *General Household Survey*, 1976, p. 78.

The rates of consultation vary immensely with the size of the practice. The higher the number of patients the lower the annual consultation rates, and the fewer the number of patients the more times the doctor tends to see his patients.

That practice arrangements may have an effect upon consulting rates is shown by the data in the next table, although this data may reflect a tendency evident at the time of the survey for larger practices to be in industrial areas.

Annual consultation rates and size of practice (survey carried out September 1964–July 1965)

Size of practice	*Annual consultation rates per person*
Less than 2000	4·8
2000–2999	4·0
More than 3000	3·4

From Wright J. H. (1968) *Reports from General Practice 8, Dartmouth.* Royal College of General Practitioners.

Annual consultation rates and appointment systems

	Annual consultation rates per person	
	South-West England	South Wales
Full appointment system	3·6	4·2
Partial appointment system	4·1	5·3
No appointment system	4·2	5·5

From Royal College of General Practitioners. *Present State and Future Needs of General Practice*, 3rd ed. (Report from General Practice 16).

C. WHAT IS THE SETTING OF THE PRACTICE?

It can be seen from the foregoing tables that the setting of a practice has a relationship to its workload, not all of which stems logically from its social class composition. It is interesting that rural practices have the lowest home visiting rates and a median consulting rate. This may be because a controlling factor in home visiting is likely to be time rather than distance and a half-mile in a densely populated inner city area may take longer to cover than five miles in a rural area.

A study of home visiting: average number of visits per doctor by type of area in the 10-day period

	Type of call			
	Acute			
Area	New	Repeat	Chronic	*Total*
Large urban	42·7	26·1	17·0	87·3
Medium urban	51·0	23·9	9·3	85·6
Small urban	50·0	32·5	19·3	103·4
Rural	29·6	24·6	18·0	73·0
Total	45·3	27·5	16·3	90·6

Marsh G. N. et al. (1972) GPs' visits: survey by North-East England Faculty, Royal College of General Practitioners. *Br. Med. J.* 1, 487.

Average number of visits per doctor per 1000 patients on list by type of area in the 10-day period

	Type of call			
	Acute			
Area	New	Repeat	Chronic	*Total*
Large urban	16·3	10·0	7·1	33·4
Medium urban	18·1	8·4	3·8	30·3
Small urban	20·0	13·0	8·4	41·3
Rural	15·7	12·9	9·9	38·3

From Marsh G. N. et al. (1972) GPs' visits: survey by North-East England Faculty, Royal College of General Practitioners. *Br. Med. J.* 1, 487.

Geography and ecology

You should become familiar as soon as possible with the geography and social class ecology of the practice area. Your trainer can describe the social class ecology as you accompany him or her on visits. It is sensible to have a map of the practice with you at all times and to begin to become familiar with traffic flow in it during week-days, and in particular at rush hours, and to know any ways used by the doctors to circumnavigate these obstacles.

You now have more than enough material for tutorial II on the internal arrangements and setting of your training practice. You should be able to use the material so that you can begin to approach Aim 1 (*d*) (*see* p. 9) of your training concerned with 'understanding of the social and environmental circumstances of his patients and how they may affect a relationship between health and illness'.

You will need to be familiar with the arrangements made for patients in your training practice. How are appointments made? Are patients able to see the doctor of their choice without undue delay? What arrangements will be made for your own surgery sessions? How are requests for visits handled? How are visits allocated? How will you be allocated home visits? How are out-of-hours calls handled? What will be your responsibility for out-of-hours calls? All these matters can be included in the material covered by the second tutorial. Forms B1 and B2 and your training agreement should, together, provide all the necessary cues. It is often useful to discuss points in relationship to specific consultations you have witnessed or conducted.

Tutorial III What is the 'Team'?

In this section we describe the functions of the Primary Care Team, the composition of which stems from the setting of the practice and relates to its arrangements and demography. (The composition of the team and its functions will have a significant effect upon workload and upon the items which go to make it up.) You will, no doubt, begin to formulate opinions about the roles, functions and utilization of the team and of its individual members.

In addition to the doctors the potential members of the *Primary Care Team* can be listed as:

a. Other caring professions

Practice Nurse	(GP employed)
District Nurse Health Visitor Midwife	(DHA employed)
Community Psychiatric Nurse	
Social Worker	(Local Authority employed)

and less frequently

Physiotherapist Chiropodist Dietitian	(DHA employed)

b. Secretarial staff

Practice Manager Book-keeper Receptionist Typist Filing Clerk	(GP employed)

A more circumscribed view of the 'Team' is often taken, limiting its membership to GP, District Nurse, Health Visitor and Midwife, with the Social Worker as a satellite. Even this circumscribed view has come under attack in recent years as some District Nurses and

Health Visitors have claimed that their work is handicapped rather than helped by being attached to practices rather than being allocated responsibility for a geographical area. It is difficult to assess the merits of the arguments put forward by proponents of the different policies. What is clear, however, is that a Primary Care Team cannot function efficiently or effectively if members are unfamiliar with each other's training or statutory functions. We would hope that you will learn by experience how best to work with other members of the 'Team'. We offer at this point some information about District Nurses, Health Visitors and Social Workers.

THE DISTRICT NURSE

State-registered and State-enrolled nurses are both employed as District Nurses. They will usually have completed a special training course. District Nurses pride themselves on providing 'total care' for their patients. They are employed by the DHA.

A District Nurse is required to undertake the nursing care of patients in the community. This nursing may take place in the patient's home, or at the GP's surgery. She has also a very important teaching role—for patients, families of patients and students from other disciplines.

Her work-load is made up of referrals from GPs and hospitals, social workers and physiotherapists, and she works in close co-operation with them for the complete benefit of the patients. She is responsible herself, with her nursing officer's back-up, for the arrangement of her nursing duties provided that the required treatments are adequately covered.

She therefore gives:

1. *Skilled nursing care* for patients in their own homes—or in surgery or Health Centre—working under the clinical guidance of the GP.
2. *Aid* for the patient toward self care—so that he becomes independent as soon as possible.
3. *Education to families* so that they may ultimately assume at least some of the nursing care required, and which they may safely carry out. This involves demonstration (including that of aids) and supervision.
4. *Interpretation* (after consultation with the doctors involved) to both family and patient of the implications of medical diagnosis and guiding and supporting them afterwards.

5. *Accurate observations* to other members of a group practice team, or to her GP, on physical and mental situations and conditions, should she discuss these during her nursing care.

The District Nurse works in a variety of situations and homes which include gipsy caravans, barges, etc. as well as flats and houses of all social classes.

She provides care for sick people of all ages who can be nursed in their own homes. For example:

Long-term chronic sick
Common skin diseases
Chest conditions—TB, asthma, etc.
Diabetes
Cancer and terminal care of same
All aspects of cardiac illness
Early discharges from surgical units of hospitals and ordinary post-surgery care
Geriatric nursing including:

1. Maintenance of health
2. General advice to family
3. Treatment of incontinence
4. Prevention of disability

Care of physically handicapped

Nursing of patients who are mentally subnormal and those who have suffered mental illness is also carried out, usually by nurses especially trained to do so.

THE HEALTH VISITOR

The function of the Health Visitor

International definition

The problem of defining the role of the Health Visitor and the public health nurse is not peculiar to the UK and expert Committees of the World Health Organisation have given attention to this. An international definition states that public health nursing is a special field of nursing which combines the skills of nursing, public health and some phases of social assistance. It functions as part of the total public health programme for the promotion of health, the improvement of conditions in the social and physical environment, rehabilitation and the prevention of illness and disability.

Definition of function in UK

By relating this statement to the Health Visitor in the UK her work here can be defined as follows:

The Health Visitor is a nurse with post-registration qualifications who provides a continuing service to families and individuals in the community. Her work has five main aspects:

1. The prevention of mental, physical and emotional ill health and its consequences.
2. Early detection of ill health and the surveillance of high risk groups.
3. Recognition and identification of need and mobilization of appropriate resources where necessary.
4. Health teaching.
5. Provision of care; this will include support during periods of stress and advice and guidance in cases of illness as well as in the care and management of children. The Health Visitor is not, however, actively engaged in technical nursing procedures.

We asked an attached Health Visitor (Bugden, 1977) to give us her point of view.

A Health Visitor's point of view

'Of paramount importance to the Health Visitor is the skill to develop interpersonal relationships; and how this is actually achieved is very difficult to define. The Health Visitor must build up meaningful relationships not only with her clients, but also with the colleagues with whom she works both in the same and allied fields.

'The Health Visitor may be placed in a geographical area or attached to a group of general practitioners. The latter I find most beneficial as I enjoy team work and the access to information about clients and the feedback from the GPs. I personally feel health visiting should be preventive medicine. The preventive aspect is often lost in the crises and everyday routine work, but it should always be "in mind" and opportunities for education often present themselves.

'Our most effective work I feel is achieved in the homes; the clinics are useful for monitoring and reassurance for the mothers, but more important they can be the signal that all is not well at home; either by over-frequent visits by the mother or in some cases non-attendance.

'Our work is very much from birth to 99, or later; and the emphasis on the whole family and particularly our involvement with the elderly gives a complete picture and insight into the "community".

'In this area we are now becoming more involved in hospitals—liaisons exist with paediatric units, maternity units and casualties and soon with the geriatric hospital.

'I feel that as Health Visitors we have a lot to offer the community; how this is achieved needs careful thought. We are being forced to look at our role. Many feel we are spreading our talents too wide and not concentrating on the areas in which we are highly trained, namely the under fives.

'We are extremely privileged in our access to the general public and we must start using the privilege for the improvement of the community at large.'

THE SOCIAL WORKER

Social Workers are employed by statutory and voluntary agencies. The former are Social Services Departments and the Probation Service, the latter include such agencies as the NSPCC, the Family Welfare Association, the Church of England Children's Society and Help the Aged.

Social Workers may be qualified or unqualified. However, the trend is to employ qualified staff and to encourage would-be social workers to undertake a training course. Most courses are of two years' duration, though there are some one-year courses for people with relevant degrees.

The work a Social Worker undertakes largely depends on the setting in which he/she is employed, and it would be impossible to give a fully comprehensive job description here. However, here are some broad definitions of the areas of work a social worker may do.

Casework/counselling

Social Workers in most agencies help individuals and families by using casework and counselling skills. There are a variety of methods and techniques and Social Workers vary in their approaches, given their own personalities and the client's situation. By offering support, the opportunity to talk through problems and anxieties and by establishing a trusting, caring relationship, it is possible to help some people resolve difficulties, change their situation or adjust to it or accept it, or encourage them to cope with problems they have previously found too daunting. For example, a Social Worker in a hospital setting may work intensively with a patient who has had an amputation to help him accept his disability and loss and adjust to a new life-style.

Statutory work

Social Workers in Social Services Departments and the Probation Service are responsible for a great deal of statutory work.

For Probation Officers this is work with adult offenders and their families, e.g. preparing court reports, seeing people on Probation Orders, helping people when they come out of prison.

In social services the range of work is wider. Many Social Workers hold mental health warrants and are responsible for assessing, with doctors, people who may require compulsory admission to psychiatric hospitals.

There is also statutory work with children. In addition to preparing court reports about home circumstances of juvenile offenders, a Social Worker may take out a court order (a Place of Safety Order) to protect a child at risk and will also work with children and their families when the court has made an order on the children. This may be a care order, placing the child in council care or a supervision order, requiring that the child be supervised at home.

Various Acts of Parliament specify a large number of other duties for which Social Workers are responsible, e.g. adoption work, the registration of child minders and the registration of disabled people.

Liaison/advocacy

Social Workers may be in contact with a wide range of other departments and agencies to ensure that clients get appropriate help, advice and information.

In some instances, a Social Worker will be an advocate for a client and will try to ensure that he gets a service or help to which he is entitled. An example would be a Social Worker contacting the DHSS to explain a client's problems over Supplementary Benefit or to explain his need for a grant.

Use of resources

A Social Worker may advise someone about where appropriate help and advice are available, and, if necessary, make a referral.

Also, a Social Worker will assess whether a person is eligible or suitable for a service or resource which is available from the agency in which he works. This particularly applies to Social Workers in Social Services Departments that are responsible for the provision of, for example, residential, domiciliary and day care. Where a resource is limited, like day nursery places, accurate assessments and a priorities system are necessary.

Other areas of work

Social Workers do not always work with individuals and families. There are Social Workers in residential settings (children's homes, etc.) and other workers who choose to specialize in areas such as community work, youth work and group work.

This broadly covers the areas of work with which a Social Worker may be involved. As may be seen, Social Workers do carry a great deal of responsibility and may well have to take decisions which have profound influences on people's lives, e.g. removing a child from home, taking a child to court, etc. The difficulty of such decisions and the personal responsibility make social work a demanding and stressful occupation.

SOCIAL SERVICES DEPARTMENT

Operational activities

1. Carrying out research into social needs.
2. Evaluating and developing the services provided.
3. Creating public knowledge of the services available (CS & DPA 1970).

4. Providing domiciliary care, protection and supervision for those in need.
   a Promotion of welfare of children and young persons (including statutory supervision of children in exposed situations of various kinds) (Nursery and Child Minders' Regulation Act 1948; Adoption Act 1958; C & YPA 1963; Matrimonial Proceedings Act 1965; C & YPA 1969).
   b Fostering of Children (C & YPA 1969).
   c Promotion of welfare and disabled (NAA 1948; CS & DPA 1970).
   d Provision of aids for disabled (CS & DPA 1970).
   e Promotion of welfare of elderly (HS & PHA 1968).
   f Provision of meals for the elderly (NAA 1948).
   g Promotion of welfare of mentally disordered (MHA 1959).
   h Compulsory committal to hospital of the mentally disorderd where necessary (MHA 1959).
   i Provision of ancillary services for the sick and infirm (HS & PHA 1968).
   j Provision of home helps for needy households (HS & PHA 1968).
5. Providing day centres for those in need.
   a Provision of day nurseries (NHSA 1946).
   b Provision of 'intermediate treatment' centres for children (C & YPA 1969.
   c Provision of workshops for the disabled (CS & DPA) 1970).
   d Provision of day centres for the elderly (NAA 1948).
   e Provision of training and occupational centres and social centres for the mentally disordered (MHA 1959).
   f Provision of training and occupational centres for the sick and infirm (HS & PHA 1968).
6. Providing residential care for those in need.
   a Provision of residential care and upbringing for children in need (CA 1948; C & YPA 1969).
   b Provision of hostels for young people over school age, who have been in care (CA 1948).
   c Provision of hostels for the disabled (NAA 1948).
   d Provision of residential accommodation for the elderly (NAA 1948.
   e Provision of holiday homes for the elderly (NAA 1948).
   f Provision of residential care and hostels for the mentally disordered (MHA 1959).

- *g* Provision of holiday homes for the mentally disordered (MHA 1959).
- *h* Provision of residential accommodation for the sick and infirm (NAA 1948; HS & PHA 1968).
- *i* Provision of temporary residential accommodation for persons in urgent need (NAA 1948).

7. Providing other miscellaneous services.
   - *a* Registration of adoption societies (Adoption Act 1958).
   - *b* Registration of children's homes and child minders (N & CMRA 1948).
   - *c* Registration of homes for the disabled or elderly or charities for the disabled (NAA 1948).
   - *d* Registration of homes for the mentally disordered (MHA 1959).
   - *e* Acting as adoption agency (Adoption Act 1958).
   - *f* Acting as guardian—*ad litem* (Adoption Act 1958).
   - *g* Producing reports for the courts in care proceedings (C & YPA 1969).
   - *h* Management of property of people in care or in hospital (NAA 1948).
   - *i* Provision of burials and cremation for those for whom no suitable alternative arrangements are available at the time of death (NAA 1948).

Abbreviations of Legislation

CS & DPA 1970	Chronically Sick and Disabled Persons Act 1970
C & YPA 1963 C & YPA 1969	Children and Young Persons Act
NAA 1948	National Assistance Act 1948
MHA 1959	Mental Health Act 1959
HS & PHA 1968	Health Service and Public Health Act 1968
NHSA 1946	National Health Service Act 1946
N & CMRA 1948	Nurseries and Childminders Regulation Act 1948
CA 1948	Children Act 1948

That there tends to be overlap between the work of Health Visitors and that of Social Workers sometimes causes problems. The following table shows topics discussed by Health Visitors in 5 per cent or more of the visits they made.

Topics discussed	% of visits in: Households with children under 5	Households with elderly persons
1. Diet	58	39
2. Development		
physical	50	—
mental/emotional	36	—
behaviour problem	16	5
3. Immunization	44	—
4. Screening	23	—
5. Minor ailments	13	12
6. Specific illness	12	50
7. Playgroup	16	—
8. School, including preparation for school	9	—
9. General health	32	38
10. General hygiene	—	7
11. Post-natal		
mother, physical	24	—
mental	16	—
12. Marital disharmony	8	—
13. Family planning	15	—
14. Employment	12	—
15. Housing	19	19
16. Social security benefits	—	16
17. Financial inadequacy	8	9
18. Household management	8	14
19. Home help	6	55
20. Home safety	8	13
21. Nursing care	—	26
22. Adjustment to illness/disability	—	35
23. Adjustment/preparation for retirement	—	5
24. Bereavement	—	8

(From Clark, 1973 *A Family Visitor: A Descriptive Analysis of Health Visiting in Berkshire*. London, Royal College of Nursing.)

You may feel that some of the topics shown in the table are inappropriate to the job as we have already described it. The result of putting individuals into a team working together is to blur the boundaries between the roles for which they have each been trained. As with any group it is the personalities of those involved which will provide the colour and stimulation necessary for them to continue to work together effectively. It is unlikely that any two successful

Primary Care Teams will have divided their tasks up in identical ways.

It may be important for you to think about these questions of role boundary. They will affect the teams to which you go as a principal and it is important that you learn about the work of a team in terms of what the group can *hope* to achieve rather than in terms of what its individual members *ought* to do.

We have provided you with some perceptions of the skills of District Nurses, Health Visitors and Social Workers. In theory there are three reasons for having a Primary Care Team:

1. One reason concerns an increase in the range of skills made available through the practice to the people registered with it as patients. This assumes that members possess different skills and to differing degrees.

2. The second reason concerns saving the time of expensive professionals. This assumes that if either of two people can do a particular job then the less expensive one should undertake it—as long as the expensive professional can use to the profit of patients the extra time made available.

3. The third reason concerns making contact with patients. This assumes that some patients who would benefit from care are reluctant to seek it. This may apply in particular to preventive medical services and examples are the use of a specially trained nurse to visit people in their homes to provide contraceptive advice or the opportunity afforded by statute to Health Visitors to contact people with young but non-immunized children.

This third reason includes therefore opportunities for what has come to be called 'positive out-reach'. Such activities raise matters of privacy and invasion of it which you might wish to discuss with your trainer or elsewhere.

During consultations which you observe you may find it difficult at first to divine the basis on which different tasks on behalf of individual patients are allocated to different members of the Primary Care Team who work from your training practice. On occasions these will be clearcut, such as the District Nurse dressing the varicose ulcers of a relatively house-bound elderly patient or the visit by a Health Visitor to a mother who reports that her apparently well, 10-day-old, firstborn baby boy is having projectile vomits. On other occasions your trainer may not delegate but make the visits himself.

It seems important that you learn about the work of the District Nurse and the Health Visitor, in the first instance, by accompanying

Tutorial III Form C

Mark Yes or No in each column

Patient	Skill required	*Skill possessed by*			
		Trainee	District Nurse	Health Visitor	Social Worker
1					
2					
3					
4					
5					
6					
7					
8					
9					
10					
11					
12					
13					
14					
15					
16					
17					
18					
19					
20					

them and you and your trainer can easily arrange for this. You will need also to look at the opportunities taken and the opportunities missed for inter-referral during consultations.

In order to perfect the basis for the independent decisions you will soon yourself be making it will be sensible if, in addition to accompanying members of the team you note during a day's surgery and visits the occasions on which you think the skills of one of them could have been used appropriately (use Form C). You will then be able to discuss your views with your trainer using specific examples as well as touching on general principles. It may be useful to have one or two members of the team also present at the tutorial.

Tutorial IV Where do we go now?

You will now be considering your own particular needs in the light of your recent experiences. Your needs may prove to be theoretical, practical, or a mixture of both. In this section we suggest some ways of learning.

As an initial action we recommend that you complete Form D, identifying deficiencies in your practical skills before you undertake too many surgeries on your own.

Contact with patients in surgery sessions and on home visits will take up a large proportion of your time and tutorials in the practice may occupy a further 2 or 3 hours a week. Plotting the remainder of your time on your 'planner' (*see* Foreword) may help to make best use of the time remaining.

The range of a trainee's work tends to differ from that of established GP's, including his trainer (Hasler, 1982) and you may decide with your trainer that steps should be taken to ensure that you have adequate experience of the whole range of a general practitioner's responsibilities. We suggest that your trainer should:

1. Allocate to you for a study in depth a patient or family who has been found 'difficult' by the partners in the practice, by the staff, or by both.

2. Identify and ask you to look after during your period in the training practice:

A patient receiving terminal care;
A bereaved patient;
A family with a handicapped child;
A single-parent family;
An elderly person, largely housebound;
A patient with a long-term psychiatric problem or personality disorder;
A 'high-using' family;
Patients with asthma;
Patients with diabetes;
Patients with angina;

Patients with cardiac failure;
Patients with epilepsy.

You and your trainer will be able to add to this list as your training period continues so that you achieve that aim of your training which requires you to 'have sufficient knowledge of disease processes, particularly of common diseases, chronic diseases and those which endanger life or have serious complications or consequences'.

TUTORIALS

You and your trainer should now agree a fixed time for one tutorial a week of 60–90 min. Freedom from interruption needs to be ensured.

The purpose of the tutorial is to enable you and your trainer to discuss a range of specific subjects. These may relate to the organization of the practice, specific aspects of patient care (e.g. bereavement) and clinical discussion. Ideally a programme should be prepared in order that some background reading be undertaken in preparation and consultations selected to illustrate them. Gaps should be left so that needs identified later can be met.

Tutorials should not concern problems which arise in your understanding or management of individual cases. These should be dealt with ad hoc *as they arise or at the end of the consultation session during which you identify them.*

1. Consultations

It seems sensible for you and your trainer to try to arrange things so that topics for tutorials both supplement and complement those dealt with on your release course. What is essential if you are to benefit fully from all types of learning opportunity is that consultations be available for you, so you can relate them to what you need to learn, and to practise and reinforce new information or ideas to which you have been introduced.

Take, as an example, the topic of abortion. It is possible that a woman seeking termination of pregnancy will choose to consult a doctor she knows, your trainer, rather than one she does not know, you. Equally well the converse could be true.

Discussion of a consultation with a woman seeking abortion could draw upon the surgery work of either or both you and your trainer and might cover: aspects of confidentiality of information; continuity of care; duration of appointments; records; ancillary staff, especially social workers; relationships with clinics of other authorities; referral to specialists; voluntary and statutory agencies; preventive medicine; family planning: . . . you can go on through the lists and select your own points of focus. It seems likely that you will learn better when driven by a need to know and it may be necessary for your trainer to try to arrange for you to be involved with a patient seeking termination rather than leaving you as a passive witness or discussing in abstract a situation laden with emotion.

There are a number of other ways in which the content of consultation can be selected for tutorials. These include:

Random case analysis
Prescription analysis
Certificate analysis
Investigations analysis
Referral letter analysis

Apart from random case analysis, the other ways listed can be seen as 'terminating actions' of the consultation and are discussed in Tutorial VI. The simplest way of collecting this information for the tutorial is by making carbon copies of the necessary material.

Random case analysis requires you to take to the tutorial all your case records from one or more surgery sessions. The totality of your actions and thought processes will be available for discussion but, initially, your trainer should concentrate upon what is revealed by the records themselves, by your notes of your consultation(s) and by other doctors' notes and the letters contained.

2. Work outside the consultation

In addition to the time devoted to your service commitments, i.e. routine surgery work, time should also be spent on other things in order to obtain maximum benefit from your training.

a. Visits outside the practice

Discuss with your trainer time that should be allocated to visits outside the practice. However well your training practice is organized it cannot demonstrate all the effective variations in arrangements which exist. You will have opportunities to discuss variations with your fellow trainees on the release course. You will be able, in addition, to visit 'special interest' practices and neighbouring practices. These visits should be planned ahead to form a coherent pattern and to these visits should be added community primary and continuing care facilities of special interest, such as terminal care hospices at one end of the life-span and schools for handicapped children near the other end. You will find an extended list of people and institutions in Appendix F.

You will identify areas of medical practice in which you feel uncertain. Common examples are dermatology and otorhinolaryngology. Your trainer can help you to arrange an agreed number of 'top up' sessions at selected outpatient clinics. In addition, if your hospital post did not include the opportunity to become eligible for the Joint Certificate in Family Planning you should arrange to attend a suitable course. You will find that there are a number of other courses which are held in your region and you should make your plans early if you wish to attend them.

b. Projects

The aims set up for your vocational training for general practice include that you understand the basic methods of research as applied to general practice and that 'you are willing and able critically to evaluate your own work'. Conducting a short project, on your own in your training practice, or in co-operation with other trainees from your release course, is an excellent way of approaching these aims. The extent to which you will be familiar with any research method will depend upon your previous experience. In this workbook we will assume almost complete ignorance on your part, introduce a minimum of language and suggest some appropriate reading.

A project should be aimed at answering a question: research is organized curiosity. Almost any of your tutorials will produce a question. If your trainer cannot answer any of your questions it may produce a project; if you and your trainer disagree about a topic it might produce a project; if you want to try something which has not been tried before in the practice it might produce a project. These three cues will each produce one of the classic forms of research project. These are:

1. Descriptive survey.

2. Analytical survey.
3. Experimental (intervention) study.

There is a sequence of steps which must be taken in designing a project (Abramson, 1974).

1. Clarify its purpose and formulate the topic. This will mean that you must read other work which has been published in the same field or which has used the same methods.
2. Planning.
3. Preparing for data collection.
4. Collecting the data.
5. Processing the data.
6. Interpreting the data.
7. Writing a report.

Books are included in the reading list (Appendix G) under the heading 'Research' which will help you to apply this sequence.

c. Other opportunities in the practice

You will find in Appendix D a list of possible learning opportunities. It is not suggested that all opportunities must be taken but it will be useful for you to know that they exist.

d. Practical procedures

There are a large number of practical procedures which can be carried out in general practice. The frequency with which these are performed within a practice seems to vary considerably. The question of who performs the procedure also varies. It will be a pity if you allow skills which you already possess to atrophy. It will be a pity also if you never acquire skills which will be useful to you and your future patients simply because you are too proud to admit to not possessing them.

3. Reading

It is essential that professional people develop the habit of keeping up-to-date. The surest way of doing that is to read but to do so critically.

A reading list appears in Appendix G. It can only be indicative but most of the books should be in the library of your training practice so that you will be able to sample them before purchasing any of them for yourself. You will be able to get a good deal of help from trained medical librarians including those on the staff of the Royal College of General Practitioners.

Your reading should, of course, include papers published in journals such as the *British Medical Journal*, the *Lancet* and the *Journal of the Royal College of General Practitioners*. It is useful to have a check list of questions against which to criticize papers that you read.

Check list for published research

a. Objectives

i. Are they clearly stated?
ii. Could they have been extended without a significant increase in the amount of work to be done?

b. Design of the study

i. Could you reproduce it?
ii. In what ways could it have been improved?
iii. Would it have been possible to obtain more information without major alterations in the method of investigation?

c. Observations

i. Are there clear definitions of the terms used?
ii. Was there adequate provision to eliminate bias?
iii. How reliable or reproducible are the observations?
iv. Are all the observations utilized in reaching a conclusion?

d. Presentation

i. Do you find the presentation clear and sufficiently detailed to form a judgement?

ii. Are the findings internally consistent, i.e. do the figures add up properly—do the different tables reconcile with each other?

e. Analysis

i. Is the analysis appropriate to the type and nature of the data?
ii. Is full use made of all observations?

f. Conclusion

i. What conclusions are justified by the findings?
ii. Are they relevant to the objectives?

g. Considered suggestions

If you were planning an investigation to answer the questions put in this study, are there alternatives under any of the above headings which you would have chosen?

Form D permits you to record your degree of confidence in possessing certain skills. It leaves space for the addition of other necessary skills. We recommend that you keep this form readily available throughout your time in the training practice.

You may find it helpful to begin to construct with the help of your trainer and the practice manager a 'book of forms' which you will use as a GP.

Tutorial IV Form D Practical skills ratings

1 (Cannot do)–5 (Completely confident)

Skill	*Degree of confidence* 1	2	3	4	5
1. Visualizing an ear drum					
2. Examining the auditory canal					
3. Syringing an ear					
4. Inspection of mouth and fauces in infants and children					
5. Taking a throat swab					
6. Examining retinae (fundoscopy)					
7. Using eye charts and colour charts					
8. Performing a vaginal examination and taking high vaginal swabs, cervical swabs, and a cervical scrape for cytology					
9. Rectal examination and proctoscopy					
10. Giving injections					
11. Venepuncture					
12. Giving local anaesthetics					
13. Suturing and other treatments of wounds					
14. Strapping an ankle					
15. Strapping a wrist					
16. Taking blood pressure					
17. Using Peak Flow Meter					
18. Taking ECG					
19. Using Dextrostix					
20. Microscopy					
21. Paediatric prescribing					

Part B

Consultations—the Largest Part of GP's Work

Tutorial V What goes on in a consultation?

The GP spends the majority of his working life with people. In this section we provide several theoretical models for studying the consultations in which you will spend most of your time. Form E will enable you to look back at your encounters with patients from the viewpoint of a problem-solver within the environment of a specified form of doctor–patient relationship.

We suspect that you will need to return many times to the themes presented for this tutorial. A first canter through the concepts will help. You and your trainer can pace that canter as you find best. In this early part of your work in general practice it seems important first to know that there are many alternative ways of looking at your consultations, then explore each in the light of one or two consultations and then return to them when they seem relevant to a problem which arises ad hoc. *You can expand the summaries offered by reading the source books as you feel motivated to do so.*

You have looked at the ways in which patients arrange to see their GPs and attempted a simple categorization of the conditions they bring. You have considered the structure, demography and setting of your training practice and also data which indicates that there are relationships between these characteristics and consulting rates and conditions seen. You have identified any deficiencies in manual skills and considered the skills of other members of the 'Team'.

It is valuable when studying anything as complex as an interaction between two human beings to apply 'a simplified description of system and order. Such a description is called a model'.

A 'MEDICAL' MODEL

You will have been observing your trainer doing the job of a general practitioner, in particular during his consultation sessions. You may have attempted to apply to these consultations what is often called the 'medical model' of complaint, investigation, diagnosis, prognosis, intervention (aimed at the removal of the cause or at least at relief of the complaint). You would have found this model difficult to apply to all the consultations you have witnessed. There are at least 3 reasons for this:

1. Not all steps are completed at all consultations to which it might apply;
2. Because the steps in consultation in general practice are often almost inextricably intertwined;
3. Because not all the consultations concern problems which can be even remotely termed 'medical'.

It is for this reason that the job description of a general practitioner includes the sentence 'He will make an initial decision about every problem which is presented to him as a doctor'. This indicates that another model, of more universal utility than the medical one, can be applied to general practice consultations.

B. A 'GENERAL PROBLEM-SOLVING' MODEL

The general problem-solving model prescribes the following steps:

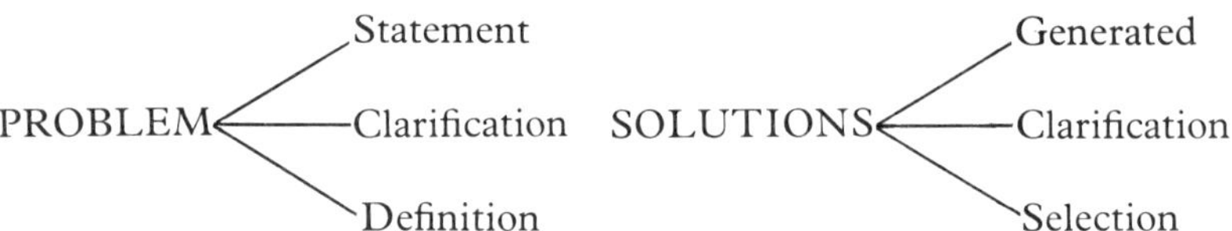

When a problem is tackled by the doctor in isolation (sitting at a desk, for instance, examining a laboratory or X-ray report) the steps listed may be taken only inside the doctor's head and it may be possible to omit one or two of them. When no patient is present, a private monologue is permissible and understandable. Some doctors, however, seem to conduct as a monologue what is obviously a duologue between doctor and patient.

C. A 'DUOLOGUE' MODEL

The characteristics of a duologue (an *encounter* with verbal content between two people) are that there is an *ostensible reason* for the contact: the ostensible reason provides an *acceptable content* which allows the *transaction* to take place. The acceptable content provides most, if not all, of the *overt content* of the duologue. There is also a *covert content* which stems from the *expectations* of the two people concerned and also reflects, as does the overt content, their *role perception*, and their *personalities* and *attitudes*. Expectations are affected by the *circumstances* leading up to the contact and by any *prior experience* each has of the other. The balance between covert and overt content is affected by the *progress* of the transaction which depends to an extent on the *style* in which it is conducted.

This very compressed model of a duologue can be illustrated by describing in the terms it uses, an everyday social encounter with a member of the opposite sex taken from the standpoint of the male. A deliberate decision has been taken to use a social encounter rather than a medical one, partly because not all consultations contain all the elements in the model and partly because we want you to realize that everyday social skills, which you already possess, are relevant to your consultations.

If the two meet at a dance or at a party then the fact is already established that there is an *encounter*. If one sits next to the other on a bus or at a lecture then the fact that an *encounter* is taking place must be established, by for instance a question such as 'Is this seat free?' (which it self-evidently is) or 'Does this bus go to . . . ?' (what kind of idiot gets on a bus without knowing where it goes?). Such questions not only establish that an *encounter* is taking place but provide also an *ostensible reason* for it and opens up the *acceptable content* of the *transaction*. The *overt content* of the transaction will then tend to continue within the constraints imposed by the ostensible reason, something about the weather, about the frequency of the bus service, or, at a dance, 'the group's good, bad, indifferent, noisy', or something. All the time there is likely to be *covert content* relating to, for instance, 'Does she like me? Is she available?'. This covert content like the overt one stems from *expectations* concerning such encounters and ensuring transactions ('I usually manage to pick up girls I fancy/I usually manage to get picked up by boys I fancy'). The content, both overt and covert would reflect aspects of *personality* such as *drives* and *needs*. The balance between overt and covert content would be affected by whether the *style* adopted was smooth or abrasive, shy or brash, self-confident or uncertain. The style adopted would vary with the *circumstances*, whether it was a pot-smoking party in Earl's Court or the Dean's tea-party for new students, for instance. If you had met before or knew each other by reputation the balance of content and style adopted might both change. Who picked up whom would depend upon *role perception*.

These characteristics of a duologue account for the presence in the job definition of the sentence: 'Prolonged contact means that he can use repeated opportunities to gather information at a pace appropriate to each patient and build up a relationship of trust which he can use professionally'.

When a doctor and patient first meet they are cast in their social *roles*. You will find some further discussions of social roles in the introductory text to Tutorial VII. For the purposes of this section of the workbook what is implied by the term is that certain behaviours are expected of people who fill certain positions in any social system. To the extent that we are familiar with a role we each have expectations of the behaviour of a person who fills that role. These expectations derive only in part from our previous experience with other occupants of the same role; they derive also from things we have learnt from a wide variety of other, more vicarious, experiences. To an extent the doctor in general practice soon acquires for most of his patients a kind of 'star' quality rather than being a 'character actor'. In other words, as a patient gets to know his/her doctor, he/she becomes familiar, also, with the ways in which that GP differs from the patient's original role expectations. This is the first step towards a patient thinking in terms of 'my doctor' rather than 'a doctor'. It may be that your own transactions with patients will be made more difficult by the perhaps unfortunate connotations of the adjective 'trainee' being attached to your job description.

You, yourself, may have expectations of the way a person should behave when filling the role 'patient'. The patients with whom you become most intimate as you progress through your period in your training practice will have learnt some of the rules for their behaviour from your trainer (and partners). You may be able, eventually, to recognize a patient's own doctor from the way you are approached during early consultations.

D. A 'RELATIONSHIPS' MODEL

The duologue model just described implies that the relationship referred to in the job definition will be formed but offers no definitions. It is obvious that relationships can vary in nature and will both affect and reflect the progress of a transaction. To that extent the doctor–patient relationship provides the emotional environment for the duologue and will affect it as much as does the physical environment through such aspects as, for instance, comfort, acoustics and privacy.

Szasz and Hollender (1956) proposed three categories of relationships between patients and doctors.

1. '*Active/passive*' with the doctor active and the patient passive: a model suitable for the treatment of emergencies such as severe injury or massive haemorrhage but less suitable for other situations to which it is sometimes applied.
2. '*Guidance/co-operation*' with the doctor guiding and the patient co-operating: a model often seen as suitable for most acute disorders less dramatic than those for the 'active-passive' relationship.
3. '*Mutual participation*' when the doctor helps the patient help himself: a model suitable for the management of chronic illness, where the patient must conduct his own regime, and also for psychotherapy.

Tuckett (1976) has proposed other categories which can exist, at least in theory: 'passive/active' with the patient active and the doctor passive; 'mutual activity' or, indeed, 'mutual passivity' and 'co-operation/guidance'.

The three categories actually used by Szasz and Hollender seem to fit best the relationship between the role 'doctor' and the role 'patient' commonly existing in our society today. There are many who argue that this limited perception of role may dangerously restrict the independence and autonomy of the patient. Certainly many doctors seem uncomfortable when required to operate within any relationship other than 'active/passive' or 'guidance/co-operation'. Some doctors seem to fear the loss of control that is implicit in the other categories of relationship and resent most strongly the reversal to 'passive/active' explicit in 'I've come for a certificate, doctor'.

Perhaps a 'control' model could be devised, although we would hesitate to make any general recommendations as to who should be in control when. One thing about control can be stated categorically—the doctor is not in control when the patient leaves the consulting room and it is outside the consulting room that most solutions selected are actually implemented.

The three models for a consultation which we have offered are not mutually exclusive. They are different ways of looking at the same transaction. It is as if they were different windows to a room, parts of which can be seen only through one of the windows, other parts of which can be seen through more than one window.

E. TWO MODELS OF 'STYLES'

The different relationships described are likely to be affected and reflected by the style of behaviour adopted by the doctor. We have said that style will vary with personality: it should be varied also in response to the progress of the consultation. To the extent that the nature of the doctor–patient relationship varies with the style of the doctor, the doctor is always in control of the consultations even when completely passive.

1. Byrne and Long (1976), have described two major styles in which GPs seem to conduct consultations. They call these, 'Doctor-centred' and 'Patient-centred'. Their book, *Doctors Talking to Patients*, will repay careful study.
2. *The Future General Practitioner* (Royal College of General Practitioners, 1972) describes a number of styles which may be adopted in a tutorial by a teacher. There are obvious analogies between consultations and tutorials, between the roles 'doctor' and 'teacher' and the roles 'patient' and 'learner'. Three of the styles in which a doctor can conduct a consultation are:-

a. Authoritarian
b. Counselling
c. Socratic

The three styles form a continuum of behaviour with the Socratic style lying somewhere between the other two.

The Authoritarian Style seems based on the assumption that information can best be obtained without the patient understanding the purpose of individual questions or the logic of a sequence of them. The patient is expected, it would seem, to blame his lack of understanding on his lack of knowledge, yet still co-operate fully and continue to answer all questions honestly and to the best of his ability. It is a style obviously more suitable to dealing with clear-cut matters rather than vague ones. It will tend also to lead to an active/passive relationship. It is likely to result in solutions being generated by the doctor only, in their not being examined by the patient, and even if the solution selected by the doctor is apposite there is no intrinsic reason why the patient should feel committed to it.

The Counselling Style requires everything the doctor says and more particularly his silent periods, to be aimed at having the patient work his way through all six steps of the problem-solving model. The doctor's interjections should encourage the patient to do this, although he may help the patient to lower defences by offering either an interpretation of what the patient seems to have said or alternative solutions which originate from the doctor's previous experience or applied intelligence. To avoid such interjections being seen as authoritarian the doctor must convey by his choice of words (verbal communication) tone of voice (paraverbal communication) and physical posture (non-verbal communication), by the totality of his communication, that this is not so. Individual behaviours which may be utilized are dealt with later in this section. It is obvious that in the counselling style the doctor is trying to make overt as much as possible of the covert content of the transaction.

The Socratic Style lies midway between the Authoritarian and the Counselling styles. The development of the problem-solving model is by question from the doctor and answer from the patient. It is essential that each successive question stems solely from the previous answers of the patient and *not* from the previous experience or knowledge of the doctor. If the doctor wishes to introduce such material, and it may well be necessary to do so, he must both stipulate that he is doing so and give his reasons.

It must be emphasized that it can be difficult to change style during a duologue: it is extremely difficult to make the change if the entire first half of the problem-solving model takes place within the environment of a relationship created by the adoption of a style inappropriate to the second half which deals with solutions.

The five models for the consultation can be collated as in the diagram on p. 64.

When a patient presents an ostensible reason for a consultation rather than a more worrying covert one the term is sometimes used that a patient has used a 'ticket of entry' into the consultation. This is a useful idea, but only if the nature of covert content is understood as something of which the patient is aware but, which he/she has ambivalent feelings about discussing. Ambivalence can originate from the patient's expectation of role-related behaviours or from internal moral judgements concerning the covert content. The point is that the patient is conscious of the covert reasons for coming. Elicitation of the covert reasons will normally be greeted by the patient with relief. If, on the other hand, the doctor helps a patient to understand an

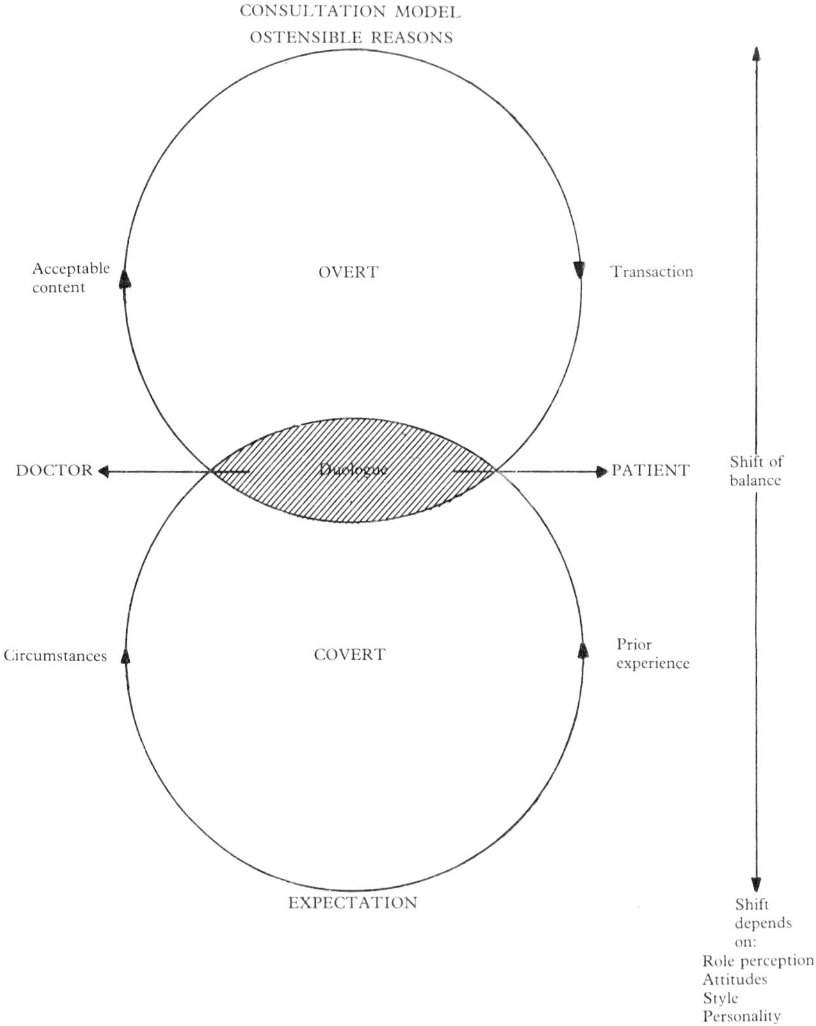

The duologue taking place in the shaded area is the 'consultation'.

association between feelings and symptoms or events of which the patient was unaware, then the doctor has gone further than eliciting; an interpretation has been made. An interpretation may shed light on something for the doctor and for the patient, but it may not always be welcomed by the patient. For this reason it is best not to be seen by a patient as accusing him/her of having used a ticket of entry. This perception of the doctor as accuser is more likely to occur if anything but the counselling style is adopted. It may now be helpful to look at the intervention categories described at the end of Tutorial VI.

We have tried to offer a first approach to thinking about the consultation. It is most likely that you will return again and again to puzzling about transactions between you and your patients. We would expect one of these models to illuminate problems you will undoubtedly encounter. The models are given early in this workbook so that they can be applied as necessary during *ad hoc* discussions of problems which arise in practice. More approaches are given in later tutorials.

Tutorial V Form E

You should be able to identify occasions in consultation sessions which you have already witnessed during which originally covert reasons for consulting became overt. There may have been other occasions when you felt that there were covert reasons which had not been made overt.

We suggest that you use Form E in some surgery sessions before the fifth tutorial. It allows you to record occasions when covert reasons were elicited or you suspected them and also to record your perceptions of the doctor–patient relationship. (The A/P, G/C, MP, P/A, or C/G: Doctor's role first: A=active, P=passive; G=guidance; C=co-operation; MP=mutual participation.)

Patient identification	*Gender*	*Age*	*Overt reason*	*Covert reason*	*Relationship*

Tutorial VI What actions can result from consultations?

In this section we attempt to tie in to the models of the consultation already offered, those practical steps with which a consultation ends. Forms F and G encourage you to record your use of these and so identify deficiencies which you can remedy during the remainder of your time in your training practice.

You will have noticed that the models offered in the previous section dealt with two completely different aspects of consultations. One, the problem-solving model, applied mainly to intellectual processes, the others mainly to emotional ones. You may have felt that not enough emphasis was placed on approaches to solving problems.

You may have noticed that not all the consultations you have witnessed reached the 'solution selected' stage. Nevertheless, every consultation ended: if a consultation ends before all the steps of the problem solving model have been completed then it forms part of what has been called 'The fragmented yet continuous consultation' of general practice. The consultation has been temporarily *terminated*, not *completed*. An example might be: problem stated as 'I have had a cough for five weeks'; problem examined including 'you are a 55-year-old male smoker and it's summertime: go and have a chest X-ray'. The *terminating action* is the handing over of an X-ray form with instructions to have it performed and to return at a stated time. That this consultation is *terminated* but not *completed* is self-evident. The fragmented yet continuous nature of other consultations may be less obvious, for example: problem stated as 'I have this terrible pain in my back'; solution selected as 'you are a flabby-looking 20-year-old lad who has taken no exercise for four years. There is no evidence of limitation of movement and your description is not consistent with my knowledge of anatomy. Your pain will go away if you follow the course of exercises I will describe.' The consultation is terminated but not guaranteed completed because no one knows what the patient thought or wanted. Equally it might well be inappropriate to seek that information. It would certainly be inappropriate not to recall the consultation about his back and the questions left unasked and unanswered if the patient returned 3 months later with a problem stated as 'I'm having these terrible pains over my left chest'. These brief examples illustrate two types of action which commonly result from general practice consultations, an investigation and advice. Until you are familiar with the whole range of possible actions and how to implement them, you will be limited in your ability to conduct consultations. You will also find it difficult to discuss with your trainer consultations you have witnessed because whilst you will know what action *has* been taken, you will not know the actions he or she has decided *not* to take. The need to make a decision arises only when there are alternatives between which to choose. Only when you are able to recall the full range of actions which a GP can take 'about every problem which is presented to him as a doctor' will you be able to fill the job description to which you are being trained by 'taking initial decisions'. It is for this reason that the aims of your training include 1(*e*) (*see* p 9) 'that you know and can use appropriately the wide range of interventions available to you'.

ACTIONS (INTERVENTIONS) AT THE END OF A CONSULTATION

The actions at the end of a consultation may be for the purpose of examining and defining the problem or be the solution selected. The distinction between these two functions may not be clear-cut. GPs quite often use a treatment to test a diagnosis, so that what appears to be a solution is in fact an attempt to define a problem, e.g. 'if your pain is peptic it will be relieved by antacids: if it is not relieved we will need further tests'. On other occasions a GP may recommend that no treatment be taken so that a diagnosis can become clear with the passage of time, e.g. 'if your pain is not due to appendicitis it will settle down without treatment'. This decision not to intervene is reflected in the aim of your training (2*c*, p. 10) 'that you understand and can use the factor 'time' as a diagnostic, therapeutic and organizational tool'.

1. Investigative actions

a. Referral to the laboratory.
b. Referral for X-ray or ultrasound.

c. Referral to a specialist.
d. Other referrals.
e. Make a repeat appointment.

2. Treatment actions

a. Prescriptions.
b. Medical certificates.
c. Explanation and advice.
d. Referral to a specialist.
e. Other referral.

Most of these actions involve expenditure of money and/or time. When considering costs do not forget to consider the cost to the patient and remember that there are emotional as well as other expenditures.

You will see that the same nominal action can be used for different purposes. In the text which follows each action is described in turn and possible purposes are discussed.

INVESTIGATIONS

It should be noted that the number of investigations performed by hospitals has increased steadily; so has the proportion of them requested by GPs.

The use of hospital pathology and radiology services in England and Wales

	1959	1965	1967	1969	1971	1973
Pathology						
Total pathology	17 279	28 560	33 360	38 792	44 661	51 320
reports ordered by general practitioners (%)	5·8	8·9	10·4	11·3	12·0	12·8
Radiology						
Total units	21 127	27 704	30 209	33 882	37 149	213 273*
referred by general practitioners (%)	9·0	10·4	10·7	11·0	11·7	9·9

* Unit values revised in 1973.

Compendium of Health Statistics 1975 Office of Health Economics. (From *Health and Personal Social Services Statistics, 1973 and 1974.*)

a. Referral to the laboratory

Green (1973) reviewed the then available literature on the use by GPs of open-acess pathology services and suggested that high-users were likely to be: young, in partnership, in a predominantly middle-class area, reasonably close to a laboratory and tended to have postgraduate qualifications as well as some sort of clinical attachment to a hospital. If Green is correct you may be a higher user than your trainer or other partners in the training practice. There are a number of possible reasons for this being so over and above clinical knowledge and experience. For instance, if laboratory findings are needed before coming to 'problem defined' either a sample or the patient must be sent to the laboratory. This seems to affect use of the services. Later, Green (1976) reported the effect upon GPs' requests for laboratory investigations of introducing a collection service for samples. Thirteen pairs of practices were studied, one of a pair being provided with the collection service. Data was collected for four periods of 11 weeks, one before the service started and three after. The next two tables show the resulting increase in use.

Average use during the 'before' period compared with average use during the three 'after' periods for both groups of practices

Group of practices	*Average requests per week during 'before' period*	*Average requests per week during the three 'after' periods*		
		'After' 1	'After' 2	'After' 3
Experimental group	73	128	131	140
Control group	55	58	58	60

The tables provide clear evidence of something you have already examined; the *process* of clinical care is affected by the *structure* in which it takes place.

It can be seen that the increase was greatest in requests for haematology and bacteriology rather than biochemistry. The increase in requests for bacteriology was predominantly for urine culture and swabs from throat or vagina. The collection service set up by Green was backed by an efficient reporting system, the average delay between sample and report being about 3 days in contrast to the

Absolute and per cent increases represented by the difference between the average of the first two 'after' periods and the 'before' period for both groups

	Pregnancy tests	*Other bio-chemistry*	*Haematology*	*Bacteriology*	*Total*
Absolute increase					
Experimental group	57·5	48	252·5	282·5	640·5
Control group	2·5	3·5	16	10·5	32·5
Per cent increase					
Experimental group	24·8	49·9	66·4	176·5	73·5
Control group	1·2	5·4	6·2	9·0	5·1

results of a survey by Patterson and his colleagues (1974) that 70 per cent of requests were available within a week. Patterson pointed out that GPs use tests for 'screening' (where the results are expected to be normal) as well as for 'diagnosis' (where they are expected to be abnormal). The next table (modified from Patterson) confirms Green's findings concerning the frequency with which different types of test are ordered.

Tests and results

	Diagnostic group		*Screening group*	
Test	Normal	Abnormal	Normal	Abnormal
Haematology	332	144	257	18
Bacteriology	162	110	9	3
Cervical cytology	42	5	186	12
Chemical pathology	120	63	20	6
Histology	2	2	6	1
Serology	14	12	84	1
Total number of tests	1008		603	

There is one likely consequence of ordering an X-ray or laboratory test; the patient must contact the GP again. Sometimes a GP will order a test not so much to get information as to postpone a decision: not so much to define a problem as to use 'time' in diagnosis or therapy.

Not all GPs are always fully aware of making use of tests for this purpose.

b. Referral for X-rays

Requests for X-rays by GPs have increased over the years in the same way as laboratory tests. The number of requests made for X-rays is bound to vary with the nature of the investigations made available. The use of certain contrast media X-rays by GPs is limited by some departments of radiology. The limitations may be for reasons of *structure*, e.g. IVPs require the presence of a doctor, or *process*, e.g. a barium enema should not be performed before a sigmoidoscopy. It may be that the use of radiology is affected also by work load. In 1973 Wallace and his colleagues reported the use of radiological services by the General Practice Unit at Cardiff. It can be deduced from their results that the rate at which X-rays were requested reduced as the size of their practice in a New Town increased.

Patterson et al. (1974) reported that 0·75 per cent of the 34 000 contacts with patients made by 18 GPs in a 12-week period resulted in a request for X-ray. Of the 252 requests made 37 per cent were reported as abnormal.

In 1979 Smith reported the use of radiological services by 71 GPs in Scotland over a 6-month period. X-ray examinations were performed on more than 2400 patients: 3 per cent of the patients referred failed to attend for their X-ray; 85 per cent of the X-rays were performed at mass miniature radiography units, the remainder at hospital departments; 16·8 per cent of all requests were for barium meal, barium swallow, or cholecystograms, the contrast media X-rays which were available to all the GPs studied.

Some of the studies of GPs' use of laboratory and radiological services attempt to examine the utility of the investigations. It is difficult to devise a universally acceptable system for evaluating utility since it depends upon the GP's reasons for requesting the investigation. It can be argued that there is a difference between the approaches of specialists and GPs to the use of investigations which can be summed up as 'specialists use investigations to make their diagnoses, GPs to confirm them'. Both groups would see as useful a negative finding which agreed with their diagnosis.

It will be clear to you that studying the use and non-use of laboratory and X-ray investigations casts light upon the process of solving clinical problems and raises questions concerning practice organization.

You should make sure that you are familiar with your training practice's arrangements and procedures for requesting these investigations: find out what is involved for a patient when you send him/her for investigation. You should construct a 'book of forms' if your trainer has not provided you with one. You will find there are many types of forms other than those used for X-ray and laboratory requests.

Try to complete our Form F for at least one of the surgeries before Tutorial VI.

If you would have ordered an investigation and your trainer does not, put 'me' in the appropriate space(s); if your trainer orders an investigation and you would not have, put 'you' in the appropriate space(s); if you agree with your trainer's decision concerning investigations then put a tick for those requested.

c. Referral to a specialist

The difficulties of classification for utility already mentioned are compounded when it comes to referral to specialists. From what has been said concerning, for instance, IVPs and barium enemas, it can be seen that referral to a specialist can be for an investigation only, an investigation which the specialist orders rather than performs.

There is an essential difference between an X-ray a GP orders and one ordered by a specialist in hospital: usually the GP does not see the X-ray itself, only a radiologist's report; the hospital specialist will see both X-ray and report. The hospital specialist will see it as his/or her responsibility to provide an opinion based on the X-ray whilst you will not have the opportunity or knowledge to do this.

Referral to a specialist may be by admission or to the Outpatient Department. In some areas the Accident and Emergency Department acts as a half-way house between these two. The ratio of new outpatient attendances to hospital admission is 3 : 2, whilst more than

Tutorial VI Form F

Laboratory and X-ray investigations

Patient identity	Sex	Age	Principal problem stated	*Investigations*						
				Haem	Bact	Biochem	Cx Cyt	Straight X-ray	Contrast X-ray	Other

one patient attends an Accident and Emergency Department for every new outpatient.

There is, once again, a certain amount of data which gives an overall picture. One in six of the population attends an outpatient clinic at least once in a year. Of all the contacts a GP makes with patients, 5 per cent result in referral to outpatients. Each new outpatient seen generates an average of three more follow-up attendances. Over a 12-year period the number of new outpatients has remained fairly constant, whilst the total outpatient attendance has tended to increase. More important, perhaps, has been the increase of nearly 40 per cent over that period of new attendances at Accident and Emergency Departments, despite the fact that the population has remained more or less steady in numbers and there are more GPs and more hospital doctors than there used to be. Whether these facts reflect patient expectations regarding a 'second opinion' or doctors' views concerning the process of care remains to be determined. These are matters which you might wish to think about and even to examine during your period of vocational training.

There seem to be a number of headings under which clinical reasons for referral to hospital by GPs could be listed. You may wish a specialist to see your patient because you simply do not know what is wrong with him: this would be a *true consultation* for *diagnosis*. You may wish to have the patient seen because whilst you know the diagnosis you do not know the most appropriate treatment: this would be a *true consultation* for *management*. You may know what must be done to define the problem but be technically unable to do it: this would be a request for *technical help* with *diagnosis* and an example would be referring a patient with a peptic ulcer story to a gastroenterologist for endoscopic examination. You may have made a firm diagnosis and know precisely what must be done in the way of treatment but be technically unable to do it: this would be a request for *technical help* with *management* and an example would be referring a patient for herniorrhaphy. In addition to the clinical reasons (overt reasons?) there are others more covert and these include: referral to have your *opinion reinforced* to the patient; referral as a response to *pressure from patient or relative* and, finally, what might be called *seeking relief*. When seeking relief one has for the moment reached the end of one's tether with a particular patient and referral will provide temporary relief.

These categories were applied to the hospital letters generated in four general practices in one week. The practices were staffed by a total of 17 doctors and 4 trainees. The total patient population was 39 500 and there were 2390 patient contacts in the surgery, 358 in patients' homes. One hundred and thirty-one referral letters to outpatients were written, i.e. 4·7 per cent of patient contacts resulted in referral to outpatients. Thirty-three letters sought a *true consultation* about diagnosis and 30 about management. Fifteen sought *technical help* with diagnosis and 39 with management. Fourteen of the letters represented the more covert reasons, 6 asked for *reinforcement* of the GP's opinion, 5 were responses to *pressure* from patient or relative and 3 *sought relief*.

It was possible to carry out this small pilot survey because, in the practices involved, it was policy for all letters to be typed and for copies to be filed in the patient's notes. Not all practices have this policy.

There remain a number of statements which seem worth making about letters sent by GPs to hospital specialists. All letters should be headed with the patient's name, address and date of birth. All treatment already prescribed should be listed as well as all findings to date. Any knowledge you have of the social or psychological status of the patient should be included. You should list the questions you are asking the hospital doctor. It is often worthwhile stipulating whether or not you are willing for the specialist to whom you are sending the patient to cross-refer within the hospital. These instructions may seem to you so self-evident that you will be surprised that we include them in this workbook. Durkin and Edwards (1975) reported a census of all case notes of patients on wards other than obstetric in King's College and St Giles' Hospitals. The frequency with which a GP letter was included in case notes is shown in the next table on p. 76.

The letters found were categorized in to 'instructions' which is equivalent to 'technical help for diagnosis or management' and 'request' which is equivalent to 'true consultation for diagnosis or management'. The results are shown in the lower table on p. 76.

Somewhat surprisingly there was no significant difference in the categories or referral by specialty.

One hundred and thirty-nine letters included a single diagnosis and 7 offered differential diagnoses, 62 made no diagnosis. In 104 cases the GP's diagnosis concorded with that eventually reached by the hospital. There was no difference in the frequency with which easily legible or barely legible letters contained concordant diagnoses although easily legible letters were more likely to include relevant histories.

Presence of a letter

	Total		*Number with a letter*		
General surgery	155		93		60%
Orthopaedics	87		24		
Gynaecology	25		13		
Total surgery		267		130	
Total medicine		112		50	44·5%
ENT	24		13		
Ophthalmology	18		8		
Neurology	11		5		
Psychiatry	2		2		
Total miscellaneous		55		28	
Total		434		208	48%

There is a significant difference in the frequency of inclusion of letters between general surgical and general medical cases ($P<0{\cdot}01$), which may reflect the higher incidence of emergency admissions in the latter. Twenty-three of the letters were typewritten, 118 were legibly handwritten and 67 were barely legible.

Classification of information

	Surgical		*Medical*		*Miscellaneous*	
	Number	% of total	Number	% of total	Number	% of total
Instruction	63	48·5	20	40	13	46·5
Request	67	51·5	30	60	15	53·5
Total	130		50		28	

In a two-tier system of medical care patients are placed at risk if they move between the tiers without the passport of a good letter. *Referral or disposal?* The value to the patient of a good letter seems self-evident. It is more difficult to establish that a good letter from a GP alters the behaviour of the specialist. Certainly most GPs have the feeling that inpatient discharge reports are written for the benefit of the hospital staff as a necessary summary rather than to clarify to the GP what has taken place and what the prognosis and future plans are.

When it comes to letters from follow-up appointments at outpatients it is often difficult to determine the purpose of either the appointment or the letter. The approach taken by Marsh (1982) would provide you and your trainer with an enjoyable, although not necessarily fruitful, exercise.

Why not look at all letters originating from consultations you have witnessed and discuss them with your trainer?

You will have noticed that some medical record envelopes contain many more hospital letters than others. Extract three 'fat' envelopes from the practice records (your trainer may suggest which patients). Look at the hospital letters and the GP notes and construct a calendar of the events recorded and present one of these at least for discussion in Tutorial VI. You will have begun also to ask yourself some questions about record-keeping, a subject about which you must come to some decisions for yourself.

d. Other referrals

As well as referral to specialists in hospital the GP may refer to a wide range of other agencies. Those most commonly referred to are grouped together as the 'Primary Care Team' but there are other agencies such as marriage guidance and special disability groups with whose activities you should become familiar during your training.

e. Make a repeat appointment

The number of patients invited to return to the doctor are completely under his control—and comprise about two-thirds of surgery attenders.

Patients may be invited to return to see the doctor for a number of reasons:

i. To reassure the patient.
ii. To reassure the doctor who may wish to check on the patient's response to treatment.
iii. To clarify the diagnosis by the use of time.
iv. To report on the results of investigations.

Treatment

a. Prescriptions

The writing of a prescription is the most frequent action taken by most doctors at the end of a consultation although individual GPs vary very considerably in the rate, the nature and the cost of their prescriptions. Research into many aspects of GP prescribing is made possible because all NHS prescriptions dispensed are sent by the pharmacist to the Pricing Bureau. The matter of GPs' prescribing has been extensively studied and therefore methods of changing prescribing behaviour continue to be evaluated.

You and your trainer will look at this mass of literature during your training year. A number of points are worth making briefly at this very early stage of your training. First, not all the prescriptions GPs write are taken to pharmacists to be dispensed, and not all the drugs dispensed are taken by the patients who collect them. A wide range of factors seem to affect a GP's prescribing: some factors relate to the '*Diagnostic vocabulary*' of the doctor (Hodgkin, 1979), others to social facts about the patient (Howie, 1974); the personal attitudes and training of the doctor have both been shown to relate to differences in prescribing (Woodcock, 1970; Parish, 1971; Parish et al., 1973); and the sources of information concerning drugs also seem to affect prescribing. An excellent review article, now somewhat outdated, is 'General practice prescribing' by R. J. Taylor, *Journal of the Royal College of General Practitioners*, 1977, **27**, 79–82.

Taylor (1978) went on to examine the range of prescribing cost and patterns of prescribing in general practice. The range he discovered is shown in the next table.

Prescribing costs were *unrelated* to duration of qualification, list size, proportion of patients over 65, total list size of practice, total population of main area. There was on the other hand strong correlation between increased cost and increased frequency of prescribing. The table on p. 80 shows the drug categories with the 12 largest differences in prescribing cost per 1000 patients between high-cost (A) prescribers and low-cost (B) prescribers.

It will be worth your while at some point relatively early in your training to review some aspect of prescribing in your training practice and these tables may help you select an area on which to focus.

It may be worthwhile also to make carbon copies or some other note of your prescribing over a week early on in your period in the training practice and compare it with similar data collected near the end of that period. Whilst the data will be affected by too many variables for direct comparison the exercise can form a useful basis for a tutorial with your trainer. Another paper which may help with your comparisons is 'Psychotropic prescribing. What am I doing'. Varnam M. A. (1981) *Journal of the Royal College of General Practitioners* **31**, 480–83.

Distribution of 14 urban doctors for various measures of prescribing cost, frequency and quantity (December 1974)

	Mean	*Median*	*Range*
Number of prescriptions per person on list	0·45	0·47	0·25–0·65
Total net ingredient cost of prescriptions	(£)690	623	286–1424
Average net ingredient cost per person on list	(£)0·36	0·33	0·21–0·66
Average quantity per person on list (units)	25	25	14–42
Average ingredient cost per 100 units of quantity	(£)1·18	1·19	1·00–1·43
Percentage proprietary/ total prescriptions	78	79·5	62–89

Prescribing and the law. You will need to be familiar with regulations concerning prescribing. All prescribing in general practice and in hospitals is governed by the Misuse of Drugs Act 1971.

The Misuse of Drugs Act

This act gives authority to doctors to use or cause to be used controlled drugs in the practice of his profession.

Prescribable drugs are categorized under schedules.

Schedule 1. Exempting schedule for drugs that can only be issued by the chemist when covered by a prescription.

Schedule 2. Previously known as 'DDA drugs' plus certain amphetamines, methaqualone, methylphenidate, phenmetrazine and propiram which are now as strictly controlled as morphine. It controls more than 100 drugs and derivatives. These drugs are marked in the National Formulary and MIMS with the cipher cd.

Schedule 3. Five drugs and some of their derivatives, viz: benzphetamine, chlorphentermine, mephentermine, phenmetrazine and pipradol.

Schedule 4. Most strictly controlled, viz: cannabis, lysergide, raw opium, coca leaf, bufotenine and mescaline and psilocin. Special licence required from the Home Office to handle these drugs in any way.

Drug categories with the 12 largest differences in cost between high (A) and low (B) cost prescribers

		Cost (per 1000 patients)		*Quantity* (per 1000 patients)		*Cost difference* (per 1000 patients)	*Percentage of excess costs accounted for by greater average unit cost of drugs prescribed*	
		A (£)	B (£)	A (units)	B (units)	(£)	%	(£ amount)
Anti-bacterial	(7A/B)*	64·50	37.50	2137	1354	27·00	19	(5·25)
Anti-rheumatic	(4A)	30·71	9·26	1142	349	21·45	2	(0·48)
Anti-anginal†	(2B)	25·57	8·53	1465	534	17·04	nil	
Anti-hypertensive	(2D)	27·00	13·01	1433	727	13·99	7	(0·98)
Analgesic‡	(3A)	25·21	13·09	3540	2038	12·12	20	(2·45)
Cough remedies	(9C)	23·93	13·24	3122	1379	10·69	nil	
Diuretic	(5B)	24·93	15·88	1532	1130	9·05	37	(3·30)
Sedative	(3C)	17·64	8·97	2993	2188	8·67	62	(5·40)
Hypnotic	(3B)	17·50	10·96	1551	946	6·54	nil	
Anti-depressant	(3D)	12·50	6·84	863	507	5·66	17	(0·95)
Anti-asthmatic	(9B)	25·63	20·67	—	—	4·96	—	
i. Tabs/liquids		(9·14)	(6·82)	(862)	(575)	(2·32)	nil	
ii. Inhalers		(7·75)	(5·92)	(6·4)	(5·0)	(1·83)	13	(0·24)
iii. 'Intal' spincaps		(8·74)	(7·93)	(161)	(145)	(0·81)	nil	
Alimentary	(1A/B)	16·00	11·18	1772	1436	4·82	44	(2·14)

* The approximate corresponding MIMS category (e.g. 7A/B) is given in parentheses.
† All beta-blocking drugs available at the time of the study were classed with anti-anginal drugs.
‡ Aspirin and derivatives were classified with other analgesic drugs.

Prescribing

When doctors prescribe Schedule 2 drugs the following regulations *must* be complied with before the prescriptions can be dispensed. This is to minimize the possibility of forgery.

1. Prescription must be written in ink—usually by the doctor, and signed and dated by him.
2. The dose, whether capsules or tablets, etc. and the strength must be stated.
3. Total quantity or number of dosage units to be supplied must be written in *both* words and figures.
4. The patient's full address must be entered on the prescription.

Registers

When Schedules 2 and 4 drugs are issued or used by the doctor himself, the usage should be entered in the practice Drug Register. This must be a bound book (not loose leaf).

Entries are made in chronological order with particulars of quantities obtained for use by the practice equated with quantities supplied or administered to patients.

If the doctor operates from more than one set of premises, a register needs to be kept for each building.

No entry needs to be made by the doctor for any controlled drug supplied to a patient on prescription and dispensed by a pharmacist.

All Schedule 2 drugs must be kept in a locked cupboard or locked container, e.g. the doctor's case. It should be noted that a locked car does *not* qualify—the case has also to be locked.

In addition to the classification of drugs under the Misuse of Drugs Act, the DHSS uses a set of categories to indicate whether or not certain substances are 'drugs' in the sense that the NHS has a responsibility to provide them to patients in the community. This leads to there being differences between what a GP can supply to a patient and what a hospital can supply.

b. Medical certificates

Doctors are required under the NHS Acts to issue their patients with medical certificates or 'Statements' free of charge when required. As a result of the certificates issued considerable amounts of money are paid to patients in the form of sickness benefits and for this reason every care needs to be taken in the evidence that is supplied. It is essential that the doctor can justify these statements before he signs the form.

The first claim for sickness benefit is made by the patient using Form SC1 (available at the surgery or from DHSS offices and other sources). No further certificate will be required if the patient's illness lasts 6 days or less. For periods of illness of 7 days or more Form Med 3 (revised) will be required from the doctor. It can be issued as an 'open' or 'closed' certificate. An 'open' certificate can be given for a maximum of 6 months in the first place. Once the patient has been off work for 6 months any length of time up to 'further notice' may be stated. A 'closed' certificate must be issued to all patients before returning to work. This can also be given on the first occasion the patient is seen and can give a date for return to work between 1 and 14 days from the date of issue. A 'closed' certificate can always be re-opened should it become necessary. These rules are subject to change by regulation. Any such changes will be notified to principals by the DHSS.

Before a Med 3 is issued the patient must have been examined by the doctor issuing the certificate, either on the day of issue or the day previously. This examination need only be visual. Often the patient asks the doctor to backdate the certificate but this should not be done. The patient himself can take the certificate back up to 6 days without losing benefit, when he completes his part of the certificate. Should it be necessary to provide evidence of sickness of longer duration than the doctor should complete Form Med 5.

The diagnosis given on the certificate should be as specific as possible. If the doctor does not wish to disclose the true nature of the illness to the patient he can then use Form Med 6 to notify the Regional Medical Officer of the true diagnosis directly while still issuing the patient with his Med 3.

Form RM7 is used as a request to the RMO for a second opinion—and both this form and Med 6 can be found in the pad of Med 3s.

Only sign the form *after* it has been completed. If a copy of the certificate is required (e.g. if the previous one has been lost) mark with the word 'duplicate'. Always use ink to write it!

Each pad of Med 3s does have on the back page 'Notes for Doctors'—Read them.

c. Explanation and advice

The term 'compliance' is now applied to the concept of a patient following a doctor's advice or instructions. That failure to comply is frequent is well documented. A useful review article is 'Improving drug compliance in general practice', Graham and Suppree (1979). It is easy for a doctor to blame failure to comply upon the patient's intransigence or lack of intelligence: to do so is to fail to meet Aim 3(a) (*see* p. 10) of your training, that 'you possess a capacity for empathy and for forming a specific and effective relationship with patients and for developing a degree of self-understanding'. Tutorial VII will deal with the *exposition*, as that part of the doctor–patient transaction which concerns explanation and advice is sometimes termed. It is important to emphasize here that few doctors seem to overcome all the difficulties of what J. Bodley Scott (1965) described as 'explaining the situation to the patient; of persuading him of the necessity of treatment; of inducing him to change his way of life; of breaking bad news and perhaps confessing the inadequacy of therapy, while at the same time retaining his confidence'. The skills required to do this are part of the skills of consulting with patients. We add here, therefore, one more model to add to those given in the section preparatory for Tutorial V.

SIX INTERVENTION CATEGORIES (Heron, 1975)

The actions taken by the doctor include of course what he or she says to the patient. One means of studying consultations is to attempt to categorize the statements or questions of the doctor under one of the following six headings, which can be used not only to study any interview but have the added advantage of providing a set of 'tools' to be used during a consultation. Understanding of these intervention categories can help a doctor keep overall control of a consultation without inhibiting the patient and they are a convenient way of looking at and analysing a consultation. Although looked at here with the doctor in the driving seat remember that, like the categories of Szasz and Hollender they can be applied to what the patient says.

1. Prescriptive

The doctor gives advice, judges, may be critical or evaluative. He is seeking to direct the behaviour of the patient. Danger may arise if the doctor starts to use terms like 'you should', 'you must', 'you ought' too often.

2. Informative

The doctor provides information, instruction and interpretation of the patient's problems. Very important in patient education but it must be kept at the right level (*see above*). Patients remember about one-third, at the most, of what they are told. It is no good them understanding the 'amine theory' if they do not remember how to take their Tryptizol.

3. Confrontation

The doctor challenges and attempts to question the patient's beliefs and attitudes. This may provide a spark that lights up the interview. It may also result in the patient leaving in a huff. It must be used in a way that the patient can handle and benefit from. Be wary of this one.

4. Cathartic

This is the release of tension by laughter or, all too frequently, crying, etc. It may involve the abreaction of painful emotional experiences. It is a very sensitive intervention but may prove invaluable in getting to the ground level of the patient's problems. It is vital that the patient is rebuilt after breaking down, therefore do not use it unless there is time for this.

5. Catalytic

The doctor questions using reflection. Encouraging the patient to self-discovery and self-directed problem solving. 'What do *you* think?' and so on. This is increasingly used in the counselling style of consultation. The danger is going on too long to the '*dry well*' syndrome. Note the value of a silence—let the patient break it.

6. Supportive

The doctor approves, validates and confirms the patient's views and feelings. This is essential for the confidence of the patient but can be over used as a 'safe' unimaginative type of consultation which is non-productive, going round in a circle. Possibly confrontation to jolt the patient out of this cosy cycle, followed by supportive would be better.

The first three of the above constitute the Authoritarian (Didactic) style, the latter three the Facilitative (Heuristic) style. As with the roles mentioned earlier, doctors feel safer with the former, more traditional approach but the latter is being increasingly used with valuable results.

There is far more to consultation in general practice than there is room for in this workbook. It is hoped that you will feel sufficiently interested to undertake further reading on the subject and to make use of your time with the most valuable teaching aid in all medicine, the patient.

In describing the six intervention categories we may, once again, seem to have emphasized the emotional rather than the intellectual processes of problem solving. Certainly, in the whole of this section we have explained clinical actions at the end of a consultation rather than those during the transaction.

CLINICAL ACTIONS DURING THE CONSULTATION

All doctors rely heavily on the history obtained from a patient. In general practice in particular, but also in hospital outpatients, the range of physical examination performed is predicated by queries as to probable diagnosis based on information obtained from the patient.

It seems likely that individual doctors vary in the extent to which they rely on different types of data when attempting to solve or resolve the problems presented by patients. Crombie and Pinsent (1976) looked at the sources of information used by GPs in reaching decisions in consultations. The results are summarized in the following two tables. For reasons which will now be obvious to you 'first' consultations were considered separately. 'All' consultations include first and follow-up consultations.

Forty-eight GPs each reported '20–25 unselected representative clinical problems'. The upper table on p. 86 shows that 40 per cent of 'all' consultations reported were 'first' consultations. In only 9 per cent of the first consultations was reference made to consultants' reports in order to reach a decision whilst 33 per cent were dealt with on the basis of history alone. Reference to their own records or to reports of direct access diagnostic procedures was needed in 50 per cent of first consultations.

The use of previously recorded data in general practice

	First consultations	*All consultations*
Patient's or relatives' history only	158	195
+ Past knowledge of practitioners without reference to any written records	38	144
+ Own records or reports from direct access diagnostic procedures	242	680
Total of above	438	1019
+ Consultant's reports	42	168
	480	1187

Total items of recorded data

	First consultations		*All consultations*	
	Number consulted	Total documents available	Number consulted	Total documents available
Own/other practitioners' records	269	1162	801	3528
Clinical pathology reports	14	209	84	1178
Radiography and mass X-ray	15	163	51	616
Other diagnostic procedures	2	21	7	96
Consultant or other hospital doctors' reports	42	1637	168	5810
Other doctors' letters	1	70	7	291
Total	343	3262	1118	11 519
Total records available (including own or other practitioners' records)	3343		11 519	

There were 13 other records which practitioners would have liked, but which were not available.

There were 41 other records which practitioners would have liked to have seen, but which were not available. Of these, 20 related to the practitioner's own observation, 11 to diagnostic procedures and 10 to consultants' reports.

The authors were interested in recording systems in general practice and did not look at the question of clinical examinations in the course of the consultations.

Morrell and his colleagues (1971) reported on the twelve symptoms most frequently presented in general practice. They introduced the concept of there being varying degrees of diagnostic certainty and divided consultations into those in which the diagnosis was only symptomatic or provisional and those in which it was presumptive. The extent of physical examinations for each of the twelve symptoms, together with the degree of diagnostic certainty is shown in the next table.

As you might expect the actions taken during and at the end of a consultation varied with whether the consultation was *new*, *recidivist* or *doctor-initiated*.

Twelve common symptoms analysed by the doctors diagnostic certainty and physical examination carried out expressed as percentage of total number

Symptom	*Number of consultations*	*Diagnostic certainty*		*Physical examination*		
		Symptomatic or provisional	Presumptive	History only	One system of the body	Two or more systems
Pain in throat	287	11	89	5	92	3
Spots and sores	182	19	81	2	97	1
Pain in ear	108	23	77	1	98	1
Cough	527	24	76	16	73	10
Rashes	302	35	65	2	93	5
Pain in chest	168	51	49	1	66	33
Pain in joints	141	55	45	1	94	5
Pain in back	172	60	40	5	83	12
Pain in head	159	67	33	10	57	33
Disturbance of gastric function	141	74	26	24	56	20
Pain in abdomen	197	78	21	5	60	35
Disturbance of bowel function	187	87	12	43	50	7

Analysis of the percentage of three types of consultation at which different diagnostic and therapeutic actions were recorded

	Type of consultations		
Diagnostic and therapeutic action	New	Recidivist	Doctor-initiated
History only	15·0	45·8	48·6
History and examination of one system of body	73·8	49·9	48·1
History and examination of two or more systems	11·2	4·3	3·2
Total	100·0	100·0	99·9
Laboratory investigation	3·3	1·4	2·3
X-ray investigation	1·3	0·8	1·3
Laboratory and X-ray investigation	0·4	0·1	0·2
No investigation	95·0	97·7	96·1
Total	100·0	100·0	99·9
No hospital referral	96·6	98·4	97·1
Referral as outpatient	2·8	1·4	2·6
Direct admission to hospital	0·6	0·3	0·3
Total	100·0	100·1	100·0
Prescription issued	75·4	86·1	59·8
No prescription	24·6	13·9	40·2
Total	100·0	100·0	100·0

You have plenty of ideas to examine in Tutorial VI. It will be helpful if you complete Form G for a surgery session and bring the data to the tutorial together with the other material listed.

Tutorial VI Form G
Doctor's actions

Patient	Age	Sex	N* R† D‡	One system	Two or more systems	Rx Yes/No	Hospital			Certificate or statement
							Consult.	Labs	X-ray	

* New.
† Recidivist.
‡ Doctor initiated.

Tutorial VII How can consulting behaviour be studied and improved?

In this section we describe some of the ways in which consultations can be studied and provide a few first steps towards ways of evaluating consultations. We make the assumption that you will continue to try to improve the process and outcome of your consultations throughout your professional career as well as throughout the time you spend in your training practice.

METHODS OF STUDYING CONSULTATIONS

Models of consultations have been offered because applying them may help you increase your skills in conducting consultations. Consultations may be studied in a number of ways and with a number of purposes in mind. Like any exercise in research or education some methods are best suited to certain purposes. Methods of studying consultations can be divided into:

1. Study of witnessed consultations
2. Discussion of reports of consultations

Witnessed consultations may be studied by a third party being present at the consultation (which may distort the balance of a consultation), by viewing through a one-way window with broadcast sound, by listening to audio recordings, or by the use of video recordings. Video-recording equipment is likely to be more obtrusive than audio-equipment or a one-way window but knowing that one is being observed always has a potential for affecting the behaviour observed. The consultations studied may be real consultations from a surgery session, consultations with simulated patients, or role-play consultations where a doctor adopts the role of a patient whom he or she knows and with whom there has been one or more consultations. You will in your first four weeks witness many consultations conducted by your trainer: it is useful if a recording is available to resolve any squabbles which may ensue concerning what it is alleged that patient or doctor said. During the four weeks, indeed throughout your year in the training practice, your trainer should observe some of your surgery sessions if only from recordings.

The emphasis we have placed on the use of recordings suggests correctly that study of the consultation by discussion of reports has the weakness that the reporter is likely to give a biased account. This is not deliberate dishonesty but the effect of defensive perception and perceptual constancy (if you are unfamiliar with these terms they will be found in textbooks of psychology). The effect of discussion is often to bring back to consciousness observations which have been repressed. One intention of your training is to widen your perceptual range. This intention is represented by several of the aims to which your training is directed including 1 (c) and (d) (*see* p. 9) which relate to understanding interpersonal relationships and their interactions with health and social and environmental circumstances and the relationship between health and illness.

Recorded consultations can be studied by yourself alone, in an unled small group of peers or in a led group of peers. You can best learn the advantages and disadvantages of each by experiencing them.

PURPOSES OF THE CONSULTATION

Up to this point we have said little explicitly about the purposes of consultation except that they are often concerned with solving or resolving problems. You will have begun to formulate your own ideas about the purposes of the consultations you have witnessed and may have discussed them with your trainer, particularly during your first tutorial.

One difficulty which will have become clear is that the two participants in a consultation may enter it with different purposes, a simple example would be the parent who complains of a cough which keeps a 9-month-old child awake. The parent may wish to stop the child and the rest of the household being kept awake at night, the doctor will probably be concerned, at least in the first instance, to exclude serious pathology in the chest. The purposes are not conflicting, especially as the parent will almost certainly be glad to know that there is no serious cause. Knowing this will not result in the cough ceasing to keep others awake. The result of the negotiations between doctor and patient may well be the prescription of a cough medicine which the doctor knows will have little effect. When there is little effect the parent may cease to have confidence in the doctor and even go on to disbelieve statements concerning the absence of pathology. The example chosen may appear far-fetched but the 'average practice' will have some 200 consultations per year with pre-school children who have coughs, not always as the only symptoms. Stott (1979) studied the management and outcome of winter upper respiratory tract infections in children aged 0–9 in a 'new town' practice of seven GPs. There was an average of 12 episodes per child at risk. Nearly a thousand episodes of these self-limiting conditions were studied. Twenty-four per cent of the children returned for a second consultation for the same episode. There was no difference in complication rates between those doctors who were low prescribers of antibiotics and those who were high prescribers. More important there was no correlation between return rates and the approach to management adopted by individual doctors. Stott concludes that 'more realistic parental expectations may be set and safe clinical standards maintained if doctors warn mothers that children may cough for over two weeks after an uncomplicated upper respiratory tract infection . . . rather than saying 'it is only a cold and will be better in a few days'. Stott, in the language of ideas we are hoping you will acquire during your time in your training practice, is calling for open negotiation between doctor and patient, for a doctor–patient relationship at least at the guidance/co-operation level, for a style which leads to overt rather than covert content to transactions, and for a working through of the problem-solving model stage by stage, even to the extent of agreeing together that there may be no immediate solution.

A second example of confusion of purposes might exist in a consultation with a woman asking for help in losing weight. The doctor may provide a diet sheet, the patient may ask for appetite suppressants.

It is a reasonable assumption that conflict of purpose is more likely to exist at the opening of a consultation than at its termination. Some of these consultations may be identifiable by your not being able to understand the rationale linking problem stated to solutions selected in witnessed consultations. There is a second possible reason for not being able to understand the rationale in witnessed consultations, or not being able to reach agreement concerning implementing the solutions selected. This reason concerns identification of the patient to be treated. Balint (1957) suggested that there is 'the presenting patient', 'the key patient' who is central to the problem and 'the treatable patient', the one who is sufficiently motivated to accept help. This matter of patient identification will be something which you will examine further during your time in the training practice and on your release course.

RATING CONSULTATIONS

You should continue to study your consultations throughout your training year—indeed you should continue to do so throughout your professional career. You and your trainer may wish to devise your own rating scales. Some of the attainments that may be rated are listed below and you may find this a starting point in devising an initial rating system. You will find that in addition to reviewing the whole or large parts of a consultation against models it is possible to look in a consultation for such behaviours and skills, the use of which are likely to make consultations more effective and efficient.

1. Items of behaviour

Being able to:

a. Ask open-ended questions
b. Ask closed questions
c. Clarify inconsistencies
d. Insist upon precision
e. Define meanings
f. Explain purposes
g. Summarize
h. Notice non-verbal cues
i. Listen
j. Remember what has been said and heard
k. Interrupt the patient whilst still maintaining the flow of the interview
l. Facilitate giving of information
m. Challenge denial when appropriate

2. The doctor's skills

The skills a doctor needs to conduct an efficient and effective interview include being able to:

a. Create the right atmosphere, to establish rapport

b. Encourage the patient to volunteer information and to feel involved in his own care
c. Identify and share with the patient the goals of the interview
d. Tolerate emotionally disturbing things which the patient may say
e. Interview logically and systematically
f. Use a style that is appropriate to each particular patient at each stage of the interview
g. Recognize when an interview is going wrong and make appropriate adjustments (any mistake in communication can be put right so long as the patient is sure of the doctor's concern for him)
h. Avoid medical jargon and explain the meaning of medical terms
i. Understand and use non-verbal communication
j. Get the patient to accept the doctor's recommendations

If you are unfamiliar with any of these terms you can determine the meaning of most of them when you discuss an audio-tape with your trainer or you can, if you wish, explore the meaning with your course organizer.

It is possible also to make ratings of a more global nature in that they deal with tasks to be completed rather than behaviours, with purposes rather than methods, in the first instance at least.

CONSULTATION TASKS (based on Pendleton et al., 1982)

1. To define the reasons for the patient's attendance in physical psychological and social terms.
   a. Nature and history of problems
   b. Aetiology
   c. Patient's ideas, concerns and expectations
   d. Effects of problems
2. To consider other problems.
   a. Continuing problems
   b. At-risk factors
3. To choose an appropriate action for each problem
4. To share the doctor's understanding of the problems with the patient
5. To involve the patient in the management and encourage him to accept appropriate responsibility

6. To use time and resources appropriately
   a. In the consultation
   b. Long term
7. To establish or maintain a relationship with the patient which facilitates the achievement of the above tasks.

Although the qualifying terms 'adequate' and 'appropriate' are included in only some of the above statements of consultation tasks, the notions of adequacy and relevance apply to them all.

In any case you may find it worthwhile to keep tapes of early consultations in order to compare your performances at different points in your training.

You may find also that you are given, or may be able to take, the opportunity to use the video-tapes produced by MSD Foundation for these and other purposes.

Form H is one attempt at developing a medical interview evaluation form. You may wish to apply it at intervals during your year in the training practice. You may find it no more than a useful starting point for developing your own schedule. Try applying it to a recorded (audio or video) interview.

Tutorial VII Form H

Medical interview evaluation form

1. Look out for occasions on which the interviewer did not appear to understand what the patient said: notice if the interviewer appreciates that he/she did not understand.
2. Look out for occasions when the patient did not understand the interviewer and note whether the interviewer appreciated that the patient had not understood.
3. If there was difficulty in communication was it mainly due to:
   a. Wording of interviewer __________
   b. Patient's level of comprehension __________
   c. A combination of the two __________

   IF your answer is (*a*) or (*b*) was that due to interviewer's use:
   a. Of poor vocabulary __________
   b. Of highly specialized jargon __________
   c. A combination of the two __________
4. Was the patient at ease during the interview?
   a. Completely __________
   b. Partly __________
   c. Hardly at all __________

   If the patient was not completely at ease, which of the following constituted the *main* reason for the discomfort?
   a. The physical environment in which the interview took place __________
   b. The interviewer's attitude __________
   c. The patient's own anxiety __________
   d. Other, please state __________
5. Was the relationship established with the patient
   a. Very good __________
   b. Fairly good __________
   c. Indifferent __________
   d. Poor __________
6. Did the interviewer interrupt the patient?
   a. No __________
   b. Yes __________

   If yes, were these interruptions appropriate?
   a. Always __________
   b. Usually __________

c. Rarely ____________________
d. Never ____________________

7. Did the interviewer miss the opportunity for appropriate interruptions?
a. Never ____________________
b. Occasionally ____________________
c. Frequently ____________________
d. Always ____________________
(*Video or witnessed consultations only*)

8. Did the interviewer respond to the patient's non-verbal responses, e.g. distress, discomfort, pleasure, etc.
a. All the time ____________________
b. Most of the time ____________________
c. Some of the time ____________________
d. None of the time ____________________

9. Did the interviewer fail to pay attention to what the patient said?
a. Never or very rarely ____________________
b. Occasionally ____________________
c. Frequently ____________________
d. Very frequently or always ____________________

10. Did the interviewer repeat questions unnecessarily?
a. Never ____________________
b. On one or two occasions ____________________
c. On three or more occasions ____________________

11. To what extent do you think the interviewer identified the patient's problem?
a. Entirely ____________________
b. To a reasonable extent ____________________
c. To a little extent ____________________
d. Not at all ____________________

12. Did the interview cover the steps in the following problem-solving model?
a. Problem stated Yes/No
b. Problem examined Yes/No
c. Problem defined Yes/No
d. Problem agreed Yes/No
e. Solutions generated Yes/No
f. Solutions examined Yes/No
g. Solution(s) selected Yes/No
h. Solution(s) agreed Yes/No

Part C

Wider Considerations

In the two tutorials under 'Wider Considerations' we cover not only preventive aspects and psychosocial factors but also exploration of the patient's problems and explanations to him or her.

There are four forms in all for these two tutorials. You and your trainer may wish to conduct a tutorial on each of them using specific case material from consultations conducted by either or both of you.

Tutorial VIII What are the preventive and psychosocial factors in health and illness?

In the first part of this sequence of tutorials we have covered ideas and facts relevant to much of the job description to which you will be trained. Emphasis has been given to the interactive nature of consultation and the responsive nature of general practice organization.

One aspect of practice organization which is not simply responsive is provision for prevention. Most practices organize aspects of their preventive care as an activity separate from everyday consulting sessions. Perhaps for this reason many doctors seem less conscious than they might be of opportunities for what has recently been called 'anticipatory care' (Royal College of General Practitioners, 1981).

Models offered for previous tutorials have focused mainly on two of the three main components of general practice care—first contact and continuing care. In this tutorial we will focus on the third component, preventive activity. We will draw, as in other tutorials, on a range of disciplines in order to provide suitable models: these disciplines include preventive medicine, psychology and sociology. The tutorial relates to the job description statements that a GP 'will include and integrate physical, psychological and social factors in his considerations about health and illness' and 'will know how and when to intervene through treatment prevention and education to promote the health of his patients and their families'.

Those aims of your training involved are:

Opportunities, methods and limitations of presentation (Aim 1(b), p. 9).

Interpersonal relationships and health problems (Aim 1(c), p. 9).

Effects of social circumstances (Aim 1 (d), p. 9).

Diagnosis taking account of physical, psychological, and social factors (Aim 2 (a), p. 9).

Recognition of the individual as unique (Aim 3 (b), p. 10).

You and your trainer may find that you need more than one session to cover the material of this tutorial.

EXPANDING CONSULTATIONS

It is now widely accepted that the modern GP provides preventive as well as episodic care. A good GP is expected to initiate consultations for this purpose. An efficient GP will make the most of all the opportunities offered by a patient-initiated consultation. There are many directions in which any doctor–patient meeting can be expanded. Stott and Davis (1979) represent four broad directions by the following *aide memoire.*

A Management of presenting problems	B Modification of help-seeking behaviour
C Management of continuing problems	D Opportunistic health promotion

Let us now apply this *aide memoire* to a consultation:
Mrs Eight, aged 38, presents, at the end of a morning surgery, her two girls Beryl aged 2 and Amanda aged 7. 'Beryl's gone bronchitic and Amanda has a sore throat. I had a bad night with them last night.'

A. Management of presenting problem

The management of the patient's presenting problem remains your first responsibility as a GP.

You will need to define what Mrs Eight means when she says 'Beryl's gone bronchitic': you may feel less need to define what she means by 'Amanda has a sore throat'. Both children are almost too lively as they climb over Mrs Eight and examine the furniture in your surgery. Both have running noses; neither cough during the time you take to examine them. You find no abnormalities in the chest nor in the ears of either child. There are no significantly enlarged lymph glands in the anterior cervical triangle. You decide both have simple colds and offer the most appropriate management.

B. Modification of help-seeking behaviour

You feel that it was not necessary for the children to have been seen as an emergency and wish to modify Mrs Eight's help-seeking behaviour. You are unlikely to be able to do so unless you determine what Mrs Eight means by 'I had a bad night with them last night' and what fears she has concerning Beryl 'gone bronchitic'. Exploring these questions may lead you to:

C. The management of continuing problems

Beryl has twice had wheezy episodes in the past year and Mrs Eight has recurrent eczema. In discussing these problems you take the opportunity to explore Mrs Eight's understanding of atopy.

D. Opportunistic health promotion

You know that both Mr and Mrs Eight are heavy cigarette smokers and discuss the relationship between parental smoking and children's upper respiratory tract infections.

During consultations some patients have a tendency to re-open an apparently completed transaction by saying the equivalent of 'Whilst I'm here doctor . . .'. Stott and Davies offer an approach for the GP to act out the equivalent of 'Whilst you're here, patient . . . '. The decision as to how far a patient's 'second offer' should be responded to is less difficult than a decision as to how far the GP should go in seizing 'whilst you're here' opportunities. It seems common-sense that patients will learn better when they feel a need to know and that this must be the basis for effective opportunistic health promotion.

You may find that the preventive model which follows will help you determine the range and purpose of these opportunities.

PREVENTION AND HEALTH

The Stott and Davis model originates from a model of disease as opposed to one of health. The distinction between health and freedom from disease should be clear in your mind as should the distinction between feeling or being ill and having a disease.

It should be sufficient for the purposes of this workbook to make the following points:

1. It is possible to *feel* ill without having a disease.
2. Whether it is possible to *be* ill without having a disease depends upon your own definition of the two terms (Is homosexuality a disease? Is being frigid being ill?).

3. It is possible to have a disease and not feel ill.
4. It is possible to have the predictors of a disease without having either the disease itself nor feeling ill (e.g. a person can be obese, smoke and drink alcohol to excess without either having a disease or feeling ill).

(A useful approach will be found in *Health and Unhealth in Practice: A Handbook at Primary Medical Care* (Marinker, 1976–81).)

When thinking of health as something more than absence of disease it may be useful to consider the notion of *disorder* on which the preventive model of Leavell and Clark (1965) is based. They divide the natural history of *disorder* in man into two phases, that of *prepathogenesis*, and that of *pathogenesis*.

The phase of prepathogenesis

The following diagram demonstrates the way the host coexists with agents which can cause disorder: note that the environment has physical and social aspects.

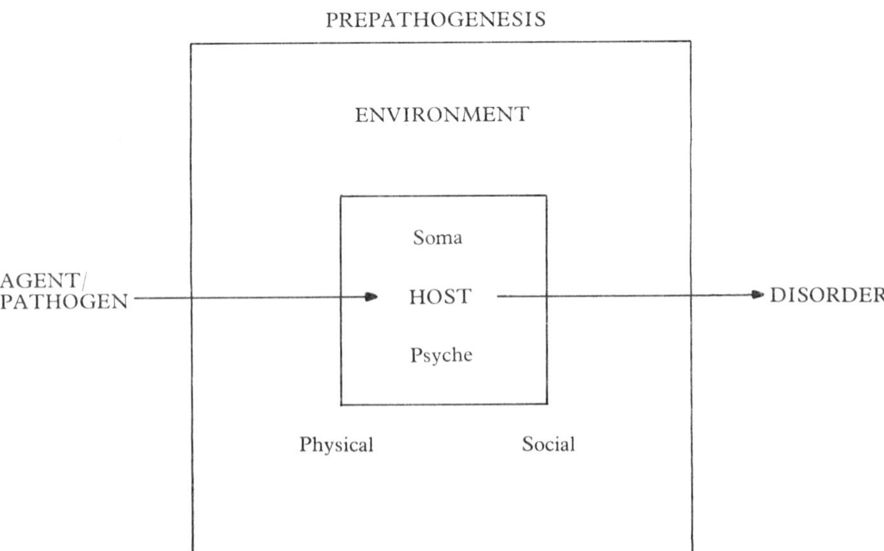

The phase of pathogenesis

The phase of pathogenesis (the course of disease in man) can be divided into four possible stages:

Early pathogenesis
Discernible early disease
Advanced disease
Outcome

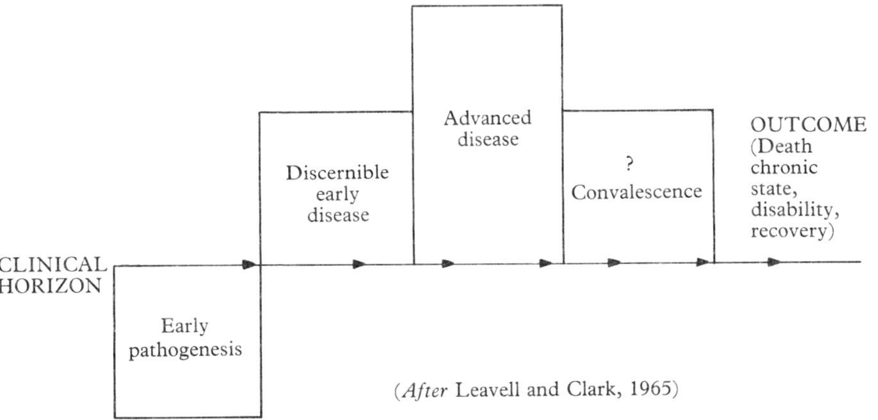

(*After* Leavell and Clark, 1965)

The model offers the concept of a clinical horizon above which appears discernible disease. The clinical horizon is the point at which a particular patient decides to contact health services. Its level varies from individual to individual and represents an interaction of intrinsic psychological and physiological characteristics with factors in the cultural and physical environment.

Unavoidably, the concept of disease is introduced into Leavell and Clark's model but its outcome is measured in terms of function. The possible outcomes include, as well as recovery, a state of chronic disorder, a state of fixed disability, or the state of death.

Intervention and interception

Within the preventive model the activities of health professionals are directed towards intercepting the natural history of disorder at any given phase or stage in its evolution. There are different methods of interception and different sizes of audience may be their target.

The targets can range from the whole world (the elimination of smallpox or the provision of a near-by safe water supply for everyone, a present objective of the World Health Organization) through continents, countries, communities and families, to the individual. The Stott and Davis model offers only a perception of what a doctor can do on a person-to-person basis in a consultation but ignores activities outside the consultation. The Leavell and Clark model allows for methods of intercepting the natural history of disease which range from changing by law or governmental action the factors operating in the phase of prepathogenesis, to altering health-related behaviours in the individual. These activities may be as important as modifying or supplementing a patient's physiological response. Changes of behaviour are achieved by *health education*; changes in physiological response are achieved by *medical actions*.

You may wish to discuss with either your trainer or fellow-trainees on your release course the size of target most suitable for different methods aimed at specific conditions.

The language of prevention

This is a language for describing the phase or stage at which preventive action (educational or physiological) may be taken.

Primary prevention is aimed at the phase of prepathogenesis.

Secondary and tertiary prevention are aimed at stages which follow the onset of pathogenesis.

Primary prevention consists of *health promotion* and *specific protection.*

Secondary prevention consists of *early diagnosis* with *prompt appropriate treatment.*

Tertiary prevention consists of rehabilitation and adaptation and is aimed at limiting physical, psychological or social handicap whatever the degree of residual dysfunction.

PSYCHOLOGICAL FACTORS

We have shown that a 'disease model' is too limiting for modern general practice. This becomes even more obvious when a disease model is applied to psychological factors. The need to consider psychological factors in general practice arises not simply from the need to make a differential diagnosis (which is the duty of every clinician) but because the GP works with people who come from the jungle of real life, into the artificial environment of the consulting room, only to return to the jungle almost immediately. People vary in the ways they deal with real life and these variations represent the psychological factors you are meant to consider.

Illness is part of real life. It is self-evident that different people will have different beliefs about what constitutes illness; about what to do when they are ill; about how the doctor will respond to the presentation of illness; and about the degree of co-operation which will be expected of them as patients.

In any consultation in general practice the doctor should have at the back of his mind a number of questions over and above those concerning the nature of the problem presented. These questions include:

1. Why this condition?
2. Why me?
3. Why today?

Let us return to the consultation with Mrs Eight. You will have made a number of judgements concerning her. Despite the untidiness of her children's behaviour in the surgery you notice that they are both as neatly and tidily dressed as is Mrs Eight herself. When asked what she meant by 'a bad night' Mrs Eight talks about her need to get up early to get all her housework done before coming to the surgery, which is why she was late and made no appointment. She adds that her husband is a bus driver who has to get up very early and gets very irritable if the children's coughing keeps him awake. You may be beginning to form a psychological description of Mrs Eight as mildly obsessive, perhaps compulsive, and that her personal resources are stretched near breaking point. This would be one level of 'diagnosis taking account of psychological factors'. At a second level you have noticed an *incongruity* between the tidiness of the family's clothing and the untidiness of their behaviour which is a *cue* to the psychological factors you are taking into consideration.

You may choose to go on to consider a third level of psychological factors namely whether or not the behaviours you have observed are *consistent* with your previous knowledge of Mrs Eight. As a trainee new to the practice you will have no background against which to judge *inconsistencies* and will have to draw upon your trainer's knowledge and his records. A fourth level of psychological factor will concern the effects, short- and long-term, of your behaviour upon that of Mrs Eight. If you decide to manage the presenting problem of the childrens' colds with a prescription you may reinforce Mrs Eight's present help-seeking behaviour. If you ignore any question of continuing problems you may teach her that episodic care is what you provide. You will be able to extend this notion of a *behavioural* description of a consultation when you consider your consultations and those of your trainer which you will witness.

SOCIAL FACTORS

An individual's behaviour depends not only upon his personality, but upon beliefs and expectations held more generally by groups of people to which the individual belongs: these are termed 'social factors'.

People have different expectations concerning the response of others, in their family, at work, and in society at large, to the fact that they are or may be ill. Definition of the precise expectations of an individual patient is essential if you are to understand what, why and when they have presented, and wish to predict how they will respond to and co-operate with advice and treatment you give. Knowledge of the group to which a patient belongs becomes therefore, essential to the doctor.

As well as defining expectations by exploration in consultations the doctor can draw upon what he knows of the beliefs and expectations (*norm and values*) of a group or groups. A doctor should be able to understand that recommending weight reduction to a member of a group which believes that a plump wife is a sign of worldly success is less likely to be successful than similar advice given to an upper-middle class Anglo-Saxon. The doctor should understand, similarly, that beliefs about the ability to control their own lives may vary with social class in the same ethnic group and he should resent neither the demand from one class for a full explanation of his medical actions nor that from another class for a certificate to state what the individual would seem quite capable of saying on his own behalf.

In this tutorial we have used already the language of three disciplines—preventive medicine, psychology, and sociology. All these are part of the undergraduate medical curriculum recommended by the General Medical Council (1980). Nevertheless, your trainer maybe less familiar than you with the language of these 'new' disciplines and your own familiarity with them will vary with the medical school which you attended. There is, however, one more concept from sociology, the application of which we believe should be explored at this stage of your training. The concept is that of social roles.

ROLES

Roles are the key linkages between personality systems and social systems (between the psychology of the *actor* and the sociology of the *role*). One individual may fill a number of roles each related to a group, and an individual may belong to a number of groups. An understanding of the *conflict* which can exist between the demands made upon an individual by the different roles he or she fills may help you understand a particular patient better. The way the conflict is responded to may vary with the personality of the patient.

Let us return to Mrs Eight and the consultation to which she brought Amanda and Beryl. As you reach what you think of as the end of your consultation by giving advice on management of the presenting problem, attempting to modify her help-seeking behaviour, examining continuing problems and offering opportunistic health education, you are in a position to identify a number of *role conflicts*. Mrs Eight is filling the role 'mother' defined by her family unit, and the role 'wife' as defined both by the family unit and the group 'bus drivers'. She fills also the role 'parent' as defined by the 'primary school', since Beryl has been kept away from school, perhaps because of the sore throat or to attend surgery. She is attempting to meet the conflicting demands of all these roles whilst being required to fill that of 'patient's mother' as defined by her doctor's practice. She has 'broken' the appointment system without sufficient reason, she has transgressed against the norm of practice behaviour and, as a consequence, receptionists may exercise sanctions against future attempts to 'break' the appointment system or obtain a home visit.

The text preparatory to Tutorial VIII is very concentrated. It is important that you try to put into operation quickly the ideas it contains. We suggest that you complete Form J for one surgery, Form K for the next one and Form L for a third. These should provide more than sufficient material for Tutorial VIII. During the remainder of your period of training you will have many opportunities to review the meaning and application of the ideas offered. Items in the reading list may help you.

Tutorial VIII. Form J

(Rate each component 0–5)

Patient	*Physical*	*Psychological*	*Social*	*Total*
1				
2				
3				
4				
5				
6				
7				
8				
9				
10				
11				
12				
13				
14				
15				
16				
17				
18				
19				
20				

Tutorial VIII. Form K

(Rate each component YES or NO)

Patient	*Primary prevention*	*Secondary prevention*	*Tertiary prevention*
1			
2			
3			
4			
5			
6			
7			
8			
9			
10			
11			
12			
13			
14			
15			
16			
17			
18			
19			
20			

Tutorial VIII. Form L

(Rate each component YES or NO)

Patient	*Modification of help-seeking behaviour*	*Management of continuing problems*	*Opportunistic health promotion*
1			
2			
3			
4			
5			
6			
7			
8			
9			
10			
11			
12			
13			
14			
15			
16			
17			
18			
19			
20			

Tutorial IX What can be explored, explained and advised?

Any consultation can be divided into three phases, *exploration*, *explanation* and *advice*. Styles and approaches to exploration have already been described and relevant notions from psychology and sociology offered. It is necessary to expand upon the phases of explanation and advice which are interrelated.

In this section of text, therefore, we turn back once again to consultations and doctors' activities within them. Over the previous tutorials you have had offered a language of ideas for most of the statements in the job description of the general practitioner with which the first tutorial material commenced. For this tutorial we have selected three of those phrases in order to give them a new emphasis. (The second statement has been modified because there is no statement in the job definition concerning explanation: a notable omission.)

1. 'An initial decision about every problem which is presented to him as a doctor' (*Exploration*).
2. 'Use repeated opportunities to explain at a pace appropriate to each patient and build up a relationship of trust which the doctor can use professionally' (*Explanation*).
3. 'How and when to intervene educationally, so as to affect the patient's behaviour' (*Advice*).

The ending of any particular consultation may be only a temporary termination or the completion of one or a series of consultations. Even a completed episode still provides data for later consultations with the same patient (or his relatives) which may concern other apparently unrelated matters. This is because every consultation provides the opportunity for continuing attention to psychological and social factors and for modifications of both life style and help-seeking behaviour.

A. EXPLORATION

If you are to learn to make your explorations as effective as possible it will probably be useful to have some ideas about how doctors tend to think their way through to decisions, using the general problem solving model described for Tutorial V. These ideas will help you also to deal simultaneously with the need to use episodic consultations as part of the fragmented yet continuing consultation which is the basis of general practice and its provision of personal and continuing care.

Early first guesses

A great deal of investigation of decision-making by doctors has been shown to rest on very early hypothesis formation. That is to say that most clinicians in most situations make in their heads a very early first guess as to the likely nature of the problem presented and, simultaneously, select a likely solution.

The most complete form of this early first guess, which tends to result in a definitive solution is pattern recognition.

1. *Pattern recognition*

You will have noticed when observing consultations that on occasions your trainer reaches a decision with very little exploration. When questioned about the grounds for that decision your trainer may have found it difficult to explain them. It is likely that he/she has recognized a familiar pattern of symptoms and signs. Pattern recognition is the result of experience although simply having the experiences yourself may not lead to the ability to recognize patterns. It may be your responsibility rather than your trainer's to help him/her isolate the components of the pattern which have led to its recognition. Examples with which you will already be familiar are the recognition of rashes or of a hallux valgus.

The number of occasions when an early first guess is so well-founded that the doctor feels able to say 'that is (————): you should do (————)' is very limited. More frequently doctors tend to use pattern completion.

2. *Pattern completion*

You will have observed other consultations where your trainer makes only a very limited exploration before reaching a decision. In these circumstances it is likely that he/she has recognized that the facts already available indicate with a reasonable degree of probability the pattern of a particular condition and has sought only to complete it before acting. An example would be 'That sounds like rheumatoid arthritis. Is the joint hot?' If the joint is hot it is more likely that confirmation of the problem as 'defined' will be sought by ESR and appropriate serology than if it is not hot.

The danger of this form of rapid resolution of a programme is that human beings have a strong tendency to value positive data more highly than negative statements. There is a tendency, therefore, for the exploration to be limited to a search for confirmatory evidence, to an attempt to complete the pattern rather than prove it is not a pattern at all.

An intellectual trick that many doctors use to avoid the trap of seeking confirmatory (positive) evidence only is to be alert to pattern disturbances.

3. *Pattern disturbance*

The notion of pattern disturbance was presented briefly in Tutorial VIII as *incongruities* or *inconsistencies*. Pattern disturbance is exemplified by, for instance, the baby who lies still and quiet when you examine him, neither resisting your examination actively nor smiling happily, treating the examination as play. Recognition of pattern disturbance acts as a cue for further exploration rather than providing a method for selecting the focus of that exploration. The first purpose of the exploration is to exclude dangerous conditions. Pattern disturbance tends to impart a sense of urgency to a consultation.

4. *Cause-and-effect relationships*

When pattern recognition and pattern completion fail to define a problem, you are likely to need to return to first principles and look for cause-and-effect relationships. This leads to questions such as 'what were you doing around the time the joint first became painful'. If such an open-ended question fails to define a problem you may be driven to go further back and apply your knowledge of basic structure and mechanisms so that you may think 'This knee is tender at the upper attachment of its lateral collateral ligament. I'll ask the patient, specifically, if he could have placed a strain on it'.

There is a need still to be aware of one's tendency to value highly confirmatory evidence. People tend, anyhow, to explain to themselves how problems arise; in addition, they tend to date observations from events significant to them for other reasons. A patient may remember his indigestion for instance as dating from a meal eaten on the anniversary of his marriage because the occasion was an easily remembered milestone *not* because the food or overindulgence 'caused' his indigestion.

The taxonomy: pattern recognition; pattern completion; pattern disturbance; cause-and-effect relationships; does not finally resolve the difficulties of selecting between the type and timing of actions with which to end a consultation. This is because the taxonomy concerns probabilities rather than certainties and does not take account of threat.

5. *Stopping*

Before ending any consultation the first duty of the GP is to make sure that the patient is 'safe'. The doctor must always consider, therefore, the degree and immediacy of threat carried by an alternative diagnosis, as well as the probability of its being present. An instance would be lower abdominal pain in a 4-year-old child. If there is a possibility of acute appendicitis many doctors would consider it necessary to institute close supervision. This might involve hospital admission, even though the fears raised in child and parents might prove unnecessary.

In a 17-year-old boy the same symptoms and signs might be supervised at slightly longer intervals even though hospital admission would seem less disturbing. In an 18-year-old girl the pattern might include irregular menstruation and lead to hospital admission for fear an ectopic pregnancy may be present.

You will only learn the extent of exploration appropriate to particular complexes if during your training you begin by seeing patients more frequently than your trainer and acquire in this way a knowledge of patterns which will help you balance probability and threat in your decisions on actions with which to end a consultation. In particular, if you decide to have a patient admitted to secure his/her safety, follow up by going to the hospital to see the patient at approximately the same time as you could have seen the patient yourself had you not had them admitted.

B. EXPLANATION AND ADVICE

There is a fair amount of evidence that not all doctors are good explorers. There is much stronger evidence that very few doctors are sufficiently good explainers. A number of reasons have been adduced for failures in explanation (or 'exposition', as it is sometimes called). These reasons have been categorized under the following headings:

1. Doctor attitudes

'Good' patients do what they are told without question; 'troublesome' patients ask questions and expect some share in their own medical management. Stimson and others have pointed out the dilemma in which a patient is placed if a doctor exhibits such attitudes; the patient is expected to be 'good' and comply with advice which he does not remember because he couldn't understand the reason for it and in any case not enough time was spent upon it. On the other hand the patient is expected to be dutifully selective about the matters with which he 'bothers' his doctor.

2. Patient's inattention and poor memory

Ley (1979) has shown that many patients have a poor recollection of what doctors have said to them and has described a number of ways in which patients' recollection can be improved. These ways are related to everyday notions about how people learn: some of these notions are listed earlier in regard to your own learning, and you may wish to apply them to the exposition component of consultations which you conduct or witness.

3. Time

Many doctors seem able to make patients feel rushed and to produce an atmosphere counter-productive to good learning—even when enough time is in fact spent. Crowded waiting room, long delays in obtaining an appointment and sheer bad manners can contribute to this feeling. The notion of bad manners may surprise you but it is surprisingly common for GPs to continue, for instance, to write in the notes of a patient who has gone out whilst the 'next patient' sits in the surgery like a supplicant at the feet of a medieval baron without a word of apology or explanation being offered.

4. Inappropriate prescriptions

If the problem which is to be treated has not been clearly defined and, especially, if the solutions selected has not been agreed with the patient, then it seems unlikely that the patient will be motivated to learn by noting the instructions given. Take for instance a consultation which goes something like: 'Doctor, I'm short of breath on exertion and I can't lie flat at night' from a 70-year-old woman. 'Do your ankles swell at all?' from the doctor. 'Yes, by the end of the day' from the patient. 'Right' says the doctor, 'I want you to take these tablets, they will make you pass more water.' It seems unlikely that any patient who is not either a physiologist or medically or nursing qualified will understand the relationship between problem stated and solution selected. There may be little or no increase in understanding unless the doctor were to add some explanation of the physiological links between the heart, the lungs, the kidneys and swelling of the ankles. In general, people are more likely to follow instructions the rationale for which they understand.

5. Complex prescriptions

Complex prescriptions of several items, each with separate and idiosyncratic instructions ('Take the blue ones first thing in the morning, the yellow capsules three times a day after food, the white ones morning and lunch-time and three of the orange ones at night') will make it almost impossible for patients to remember what to do even though each bottle of tablets should have the precise instructions written on its label.

A number of suggestions have been made as to ways of tackling the problems of advising. These include:

a. The use of explicit categorization
b. The use of written instructions
c. The use of tape-recordings
d. The use of feed-back
e. Careful supervision

f. Gadgets
g. Clarification of conflicting explanations

a. Explicit categorization

This involves telling the patient the headings of what you will be telling him, arranging your instructions under those headings, and then repeating them. An example would refer to a 70-year-old lady complaining of dyspnoea.

> 'I am going to give you three different sorts of tablets. White ones to make you pass more water, blue ones to strengthen your heart, and yellow shiny ones which replace a substance that passes out of your body because you are passing more water.
>
> 'I want you to take one of each tablet in the morning. At 1.00 p.m. I want you to take one white water tablet and one yellow replacement tablet. Before you go to bed one blue heart tablet and one yellow replacement tablet.
>
> 'Here is a written chart of the tablets. You see that altogether you take two water tablets a day, two heart tablets a day, and three replacement tablets a day. Any of these tablets due at the same time can be taken together.
>
> 'I have given you a lot of instructions and you may be unable to remember all I have said. Would you try to tell me what tablets you should take when and what the purpose of each is. Do look at the chart if you wish.'

This may seem a lengthy way of giving instructions. It will be worthwhile if your patients keep to their treatment. On the other hand even if the instructions *are* remembered patients may not comply with their treatment unless they understand the purpose of doing so at a more detailed level than 'these will make you feel better'. After all, if the white water tablets are frusemide your patient will be socially inconvenienced by the need to be near a W.C. for 8 hours a day! The matter of more detailed explanations will be dealt with under the heading 'Spiels' on p. 121.

b. Written instructions

These are sometimes better tailored to the individual patient, as in the example above, or you may prefer to use prepared sets of instructions.

Some drug companies provide printed pads of simple instructions. We do not wish to discourage you from using them but would encourage you to be quite sure, first that they say precisely what you want them to, and second, that they do not recommend the use of any branded goods. We would remind you, also that there are some indications that patients are more likely to obey instructions signed by their own doctor on his own notepaper.

c. *Tape-recordings*

These have advantages in that the patient can take them away and listen to them as often as wished: they have the disadvantage that they cannot be asked questions. The matter of whose voice is on the tape should be considered in the same way as you were asked to think about from whom written instructions should appear to originate. The tapes can be listened to with relatives and then points can be discussed later with the doctor.

d. *Immediate feedback*

Immediate feedback is limited by written or tape-recorded instructions and facilitated by verbal ones. You should remember this and check upon understanding as well as on compliance when the patient attends for review or repeat prescription. If your trainer uses some form of repeat prescription card you should not issue such a card until you are satisfied that the patient has comprehended and remembered the instructions and purpose of the prescription, that he or she can carry out any of the manual operations necessary (use a spinhaler or aerosol for instance). Further, you should check whether or not the repeat prescription system is monitored to check that there is compliance.

e. *Careful supervision*

The need for careful supervision and some methods of conducting it have just been outlined. You will no doubt think of others.

f. Gadgets

Gadgets such as pill-boxes with compartments (Pillsure, Dosett, Mediset, Medidos) may help patients who are on long-term medication. Pre-packaging of the type used for the combined contraceptive pill can be used to similar advantage with the added benefit of reducing the risks of accidental ingestion by children.

g. Clarification of conflicting explanations

The need to clarify conflicting explanations is self-evident, as should by now be the need to elicit such conflicts from the patient. Conflicting explanations can originate in lack of clarity on the part of the doctor, lack of comprehension on the part of the patient, or lack of communication between different caring agencies. Lack of clarity is, of course, linked with lack of comprehension. Clarity of explanation can be improved if the doctor takes the opportunity to polish his explanations, to develop 'spiels'.

'Spiels' You will find that there are a number of conditions which require you to be able to explain to the patient in simple terms, medical concepts which are complex and usually couched in jargon. Two examples where compliance is involved might be rhesus incompatibility and fissure-in-ano. You will be able to think of many others. Two examples where decisions are involved might be: alphafetoprotein testing in a pregnant woman and contraception. Since these explanations are needed on a number of occasions it seems sensible to be aware that you make them, and to develop them over the years so as to increase their effectiveness. We enter two caveats: one, you may need to adjust these polished explanations for different patients; two, you should ask the patient 'Shall I give you my routine piece about . . . (e.g. fissure-in-ano) . . . and then we can discuss your decision'.

We feel that it will be less than helpful to provide you with a standard 'spiel', even for those conditions we have given as examples. We suggest that you should prepare a 'spiel' for a condition you have identified during a consultation session as requiring one. This prepared explanation should be brought to a tutorial and discussed with your trainer.

Try completing Form M during one of the consultation sessions between Tutorials VIII and IX. It will help if you have also one prepared 'spiel' later for discussion with your trainer. This discussion will be even more valuable if you have managed to record the salient points of one of your trainer's 'spiels'.

Tutorial IX Form M

Ring one of the initials under each of exploration, explanation and advice.

Exploration: R=pattern recognition; C=pattern completion; D=pattern disturbance; E=cause and effect relationships.

Explanation: O=no explanation given; U=explanation given and understanding checked; NU=explanation given but understanding not checked.

Advice: O=no advice given; EC=advice explicit categorization; A=advice without categorization.

Patient No.	*EXPLORATION (Method of diagnosis)*	*EXPLANATION (spiel)*	*ADVICE (use of explicit categorization)*
	R C D E	O U NU	O EC A
	R C D E	O U NU	O EC A
	R C D E	O U NU	O EC A
	R C D E	O U NU	O EC A
	R C D E	O U NU	O EC A
	R C D E	O U NU	O EC A
	R C D E	O U NU	O EC A
	R C D E	O U NU	O EC A
	R C D E	O U NU	O EC A
	R C D E	O U NU	O EC A

CODA

Models are as useful as you find them to be. To some people models are instructional toys to play with; for other people models represent a miniature version of reality. Do not reject any of the models we have offered before you have attempted to play with them.

Appendix A Trainee contract

All employees are required by law to have a contract and trainees are no exception.

A model contract between trainer and trainee has been composed by the General Medical Services Committee and is available to members from the British Medical Association. The purpose of such a contract is to define the responsibilities and duties of both trainer and trainee to avoid dispute both during the training period and after it has finished.

The points which should be covered in such a contract can be listed under various headings.

General

Dates of training period
Length of notice for termination
Salary and allowances
Membership of a Medical Defence Organization
Fees paid to trainer
Hours of work

Leave

Holiday and sundry leave
Sickness
Maternity leave

Duties and Responsibilities

Telephone
'Back-up cover' for trainee
Equipment
Work outside the practice
Records
Confidentiality

Residence of trainee
Provision of adequate transport

Miscellaneous

Treatment of patients of the practice after end of training period
Procedure for disputes

Appendix B Practice finance

Until he enters general practice, the trainee will have had little or no experience of seeing the practice of medicine linked to the aspect of running a business. There is no doubt that the doctor who is aware of the business potential of his practice will earn more money than the one who is not so motivated.

Most practice agreements made between the partners in a practice stipulate that all the money earned in the course of their professional work shall be paid into the practice account (sometimes minor exceptions are made to this by agreement between the partners). Usually the trainee is expected to see that fees due to him are collected conscientiously and paid into the practice account also.

Money enters the practice from different sources:

1. National Health Service.
2. Income from Private Patients (in effect only providing a small amount of income in most practices).
3. Certification and reports—for which a fee is paid
   a. Insurance examinations and reports
   b. Other medical examinations and certificates
   c. Legal reports
   d. Cremation fees.
4. Income from appointments outside the practice
   a. Appointments with local authorities
   b. Hospital appointments
   c. Part time appointments to industries and schools
   d. Teaching and lecturing.

The income received from most of these sources is self-explanatory. That, however, received from the National Health Service is very complicated, and will now be described in broad outlines.

Detailed information on the way a doctor is paid by the Family Practitioner Committee can be obtained from the *Red Book* (the Statement of Fees and Allowances payable to General Practitioners in England and Wales) a copy of which should have been issued to the trainee after his appointment into practice.

Trainees are invited to complete payment details using the *Red Book* for up-to-date information.

I. *Fixed Payments*

a. Basic Practice Allowance—when paid in full £ ______________

b. Supplementary Practice Allowance for out of hours responsibilities. Full rate if more than 1000 patients £ ______________

II. *Fees only Payable when Relevant Forms Completed*

A. *Capitation Fee*—Annual fee paid by quarterly instalments only after patient has registered with the practice

a. Under 65 years £ ______________

b. 65–74 years £ ______________

c. 75 + years £ ______________

Supplementary Capitation Fee is also paid for out of hours service for each patient in excess of 1000 £ ______________

B. *Temporary Resident Fee* up to £ ______________

C. *Items of Service Fees*

a. Contraceptive Fee

i. Ordinary—OCP, Cap, IUCD check £ ______________

ii. Intrauterine device fee £ ______________

iii. Annual follow-up fee £ ______________

b. Vaccination and Immunization £ ______________

c. Cervical cytology £ ______________

d. Night visit fee (11 p.m.–7.00 a.m.) £ ______________

e. Maternity services and miscarriage, full care and delivery £ ______________

f. Arrest of dental haemorrhage £ ______________

g. Emergency treatment fee £ ______________

h. Anaesthetic fee up to £ ______________

III. *Fees based on GP Qualifications*

A. Vocational Training Allowance £ ______________

B. Seniority Allowance

First payment (years) £ ______________

Second payment (years) £ ______________

Third payment (years) £ ______________

C. Postgraduate Training Allowance £ ______________

D. GP Trainer Allowance £ ____________
(In addition to this amount a car allowance of £_______ is paid for the trainee.)

IV. *Fees for Type or Position of Practice*

A. Group Practice Allowance—where three or more doctors are practising in close association with each other £ ____________

B. Rural Practice Payments £ ____________

C. Dispensing Fee £ ____________

D. Designated Area Allowance £ ____________

E. Initial Practice Allowance £ ____________

F. Inducement Allowance £ ____________

V. *Reimbursements*

A. Rental on Premises
Health centre
Privately rented premises
Notional, i.e. where owner occupied premises

B. Direct Reimbursement of employed staff—up to 70 per cent of total salary. (Each doctor is entitled to employ two full-time staff or equivalent.)

In the past year 1975–76 the proportion of income received from the National Health Service as a national average was:

Fixed sum	21%
Capitation	45%
Item of Service	6%
GP qualifications	6%
Premises	12%

The FPC pays the doctors in their area three months in arrears. It is possible for the doctors to receive a proportion of their quarterly payments each month—which can be beneficial from the point of view of 'cash flow'.

In addition to the above amounts of money, the training practice receives from the FPC the full salary of the trainee. This also is paid in the quarterly cheque—three months in arrears!

The total amount of money entering the practice from any source is termed the 'gross income' and it is from this money that the partners receive their income and the practice runs.

Depending on the amount of work undertaken by the partners, and the efficiency with which claims are made, the annual gross income received by the practice can be in the region of £30 000 for each partner. In a large practice of several doctors this can amount to a considerable amount of money and it is thus essential to see that the book-keeping in the practice is methodical and reliable, and that a competent accountant is appointed who can advise the practice on financial and tax matters and prepare the annual Balance Sheet.

The total 'gross income' is divided into two:

A. *Practice Expenses*

i. Capital Expenses
- New equipment and furniture
- New buildings

ii. Running Expenses

a. Health Centre

Consolidated service charge levied by DHA and deducted quarterly from the payments to the doctors to cover the costs in the Health Centre including staff. The doctor has responsibility for paying personal staff, and his trainee.

b. Private Premises

Staff costs, including trainee
- Wages
- NHI

Cost of Premises
- Rent
- Rates
- Repairs/redecorations
- Insurance

Servicing Costs
- Telephones
- Heat and light
- Postage, stationery
- Printing

Professional costs
- Accountancy
- Legal costs
- Bank charges
- Subscriptions
- Professional insurance
- Books and journals

B. *Net Profit*

The money remaining in the practice after all expenses have been paid is known as the 'net profit' and it is this sum that is divided between the partners.

In the past the senior partner in the practice took a larger share of 'the cake' than the other partners, but nowadays where partners are undertaking similar workloads 'parity' is usually received within a few years.

When a new partner enters a practice he usually works for a smaller percentage in the early days while he becomes established. It is expected that the longer he is in the practice the greater his contribution to the income of that practice and parity may well be reached within 2, 3 or 4 years of joining according to the partnership agreement which should be drawn up before the new doctor enters the practice.

It is the total net profit of the practice which is assessed for income tax purposes—and the inspectors make their tax assessment on this amount of money. The individual tax liability for each of the partners is allocated by the accountant. This tax is collected from the partnership—one year in arrears—thus a new partner may have little or nothing to pay in the way of tax in his first year of practice, the snag being that when he eventually leaves a practice he may have to meet a large tax demand one year later!

Different practices have different ways of withdrawing money from the practice. Some may take monthly or quarterly cheques. Others may take money out when it is required. In all cases an adjustment can be made when the accountant has drawn up the balance sheet.

It will be appreciated that the partners will usually be expected to leave a certain amount of money in the practice for the day-to-day running of the business.

When a new partner joins a practice the payment of any form of 'goodwill' is illegal. He may be required to buy his share of the practice building where the practice is run from premises owned by the partners—but even here it is required that an independent valuer is called to assess the true value of the property to avoid the possibility of 'goodwill' being hidden in the capital the doctor is asked to provide.

Appendix C Record systems

You should know that there have been a series of suggestions concerning size of record and type of record card.

The A4 system, as its name indicates, is similar in format to a hospital recording system. The problems it poses concern the cost of converting and re-converting the present medical record envelopes.

There are at least two systems based on the present-sized medical record envelope.

The Aldeburgh Record System was described in the *British Medical Journal*, 10 September 1977 by Dr Ian Tait. It employs some six different specially printed cards. The first is a medical summary card, the back of which provides a record of the immunization state, basic physical findings and background information. Card 2 is a family and personal history card. Card 3 is a drug treatment card. A separate card is used for repeat prescriptions, while a multipurpose flow sheet aids the follow-up of patients with conditions requiring long-term management.

To these can be added a simple patient questionnaire to provide a data base. In addition, cards are used for recording day-to-day notes. This system can either be used with standard medical envelopes or A4 folders—and it is necessary to purchase the cards in order to make the system work.

The Crediton system of records was described by Christopher Maycock in the *British Medical Journal*, 25 November 1978, and seems to be one of the most practical methods of note-keeping described so far for the service GP to use.

This system uses overprinting of record cards already supplied by the DHSS—to produce three special purpose cards which are attached to the front of the continuation cards. The continuation cards are arranged to read like a book with the most recent cards at the back. The first special purpose card is for repeat prescriptions; the second is the immunization card as already supplied, with the back used as a general purpose flow chart; the third is a problem list; the fourth is a continuation card overprinted with the title 'Patient Profile' which contains the 'family tree'—originally described by J. C. C. Cormack in 1975 (*J. R. Coll. Gen. Pract.*).

Diagnosis or analysis of the problem is highlighted on the continuation cards by drawing a rectangle round it.

The Crediton system is not as sophisticated as some systems that have been described and it is for that very reason that it could well become a system which is acceptable to most GPs—for not only is it simple to use but the cost involved is minimal.

COMPUTER SYSTEMS

You will have been aware of discussion focused on the use of computers in general practice. You will find 'Computers in Primary Care'—Occasional Paper No. 13, published by the *Journal of the Royal College of General Practitioners*, a good source of ideas concerning the relevance of computer systems to general practice. However effective these systems may become they will always depend upon the quality of information input to them and in this sense are no more than technological, as opposed to conceptual, advances in record keeping.

A PROBLEM-ORIENTATED RECORD SYSTEM

There is a good deal of literature on the subject of problem-orientated medical records (POMR). This workbook is not the place to review it. It is probably worthwhile, however, to review briefly the components of POMR and the basic principles on which the system is based.

The underlying notion is that action should only be taken at the level to which a patient's problem(s) have been defined and that such definition is related directly to the degree to which all relevant information is available. The detailed anatomy of POMR can be varied according to the place it is kept and the purposes to which the information will be put; it is the physiology of the system that matters.

The essential components of POMR

A data base—this includes relatively 'fixed data' such as name, address, occupation, marital status. It includes also past medical history, and facts about the family and housing.

A problem list—this is written at the doctor's 'true level of understanding' so that 'unexplained chest pain' is recorded as such rather than '? myocardial infarction'. Social problems can also be recorded so that 'wife died three months ago' is recorded rather than '?bereavement reaction'.

Problems are categorized as 'active' or 'inactive'. When problems are removed or resolved they are transferred to the data base. The problems are given numbers.

Treatment sheet

This records medicine, advice and agencies directed to helping the patient with problems listed. Treatments can be coded by number to the problems at which they are directed.

Clinical notes

These record the present and recent contacts with the patient. They are often recorded under the following sub-headings which form the mnemonic SOAPITE.

1. '*S*' *subjective*. The patient's symptoms or complaints, their duration, the relation and order of onset and the patient's own assessment of them; associated family or environmental information and relevant information regarding the patient's past medical history.
2. '*O*' *objective*. The physician's physical examination of the patient and the results of any immediate investigation in the consulting room.
3. '*A*' *assessment*. The interpretation of the data in physical, psychological and social terms. This may be a definitive diagnosis or a differential diagnosis. Where the data do not permit either of these, the problem may be stated in descriptive terms. A descriptive statement is particularly appropriate in the case of psychosocial problems, where a nomenclature has yet to be defined.
4. '*P*' *plan*. A statement of the clinical management plan.

The clinical management plan

You will have realized already that a consultation may be divided into two sections, the first part, already described, is to identify the patient's problem or problems, and the second is to take a management decision. We accept that a solution which clears up the problem may not be possible at every first consultation and, indeed, the nature of the problem may be such that it can only be partly solved.

The clinical management plan has been divided by Dr H. W. Acheson into the following parts:

5. *'I' information.* This includes:

a. Obtaining further information from the patient's relatives, previous notes, other members of the health care team and any other source.

b. Further information which may be obtained from a study of the natural history of the problem or disease and its response to treatment.

c. Investigations either to confirm a probable diagnosis, to establish a precise diagnosis or to exclude an improbable diagnosis. Such investigations may include the establishment of base-line data which will be required for the management of the problem and may include criteria for action. For example, 'if the blood sugar drops below "X" mmol/l, then . . .'.

6. *'T' therapy.* This includes not only such things as treatment, drugs and physiotherapy, but also advice on diet, social or environmental change. (These are transferred like the problem to the appropriate parts of the record.)

7. *'E' education.* This includes the explanation and prognosis given to the patient about his problem or disease and what the doctor says he intends to do in the way of treatment or investigation.

Appendix D Some possible learning opportunities

The trainee will, of course, do surgery sessions and visits on his own.

In the Practice the trainee can:
- Sit in the waiting room
- Help in the reception area
- Work with: Practice Nurse, District Nurse, Health Visitor, Social Worker

Sit in with each partner in turn
- Help with: antenatal clinic, development clinic, immunization clinic, well-woman clinic, hypertension clinic, geriatric clinic, obesity clinic, as and if the practice (or neighbouring practices) conduct them

Associated with the Practice the trainee can:
- Talk with the local pharmacist
- Follow-up patients sent to hospital
- Go on a domiciliary visit with a consultant
- Go with patient in ambulance to hospital
- Attend practice business meetings
- Attend practice-based continuing education

With his Trainer the trainee can:
- Sit in on surgery sessions
- Have trainer sit in on his surgery sessions
- Accompany trainer on visits
- Have *ad hoc*, problem-related, discussions
- Have tutorials based on: the workbook, random case analyses, set topics, copies of referral letters, copies of EC 10a, review of pathology and X-ray requests, letters and reports from hospital, review of complete surgery audio or video-tape consultation analyses, role play, simulated patient, problem-orientated medical record, designing an algorithm
- Accompany trainer to committees

Outside the Practice the trainee can:
- Attend a release course
- Attend course in contraception
- Attend selected outpatient sessions

Attend other selected and focused courses, e.g. in developmental assessment
Attend case conferences of any kind
Attend committee meetings of LMC, BMA, RCGP as observer
Read

In Association with Course Organizer and Trainer the trainee can:
Undertake visits to suitable facilities, e.g. factory, occupational health service, residential homes
Undertake a project which may be audit or research
Swap practices with another trainee for a short period of time
Visit other practices

Appendix E Day release topics*

Topics covered in over 75 per cent of areas

The structure of general practitioner services (Department of Health and Social Security; Scottish Home and Health Department; Family Practitioner Committee, etc.)
The Community Nurse
The Health Visitor
Social work
The Membership examination of the Royal College of General Practitioners; multiple choice and modified essay questions
Terminal care/bereavement

Topics covered in 50–74 per cent of areas

Prescribing in general practice
Medicolegal aspects
Finance
Records in general practice
Old age
Family planning
Psychosexual difficulties
Child development/assessment
Skin disorders
Eye disorders

Topics covered in 25–49 per cent of areas

The consultation
Research
Problem solving
Choosing a practice
Practice administration
The Regional Medical Officer
Chronic disability/handicap
Adolescence
Alcoholism
Marriage guidance
Abortion
Asthma
The doctor's bag

*Howie J. G. R. (1977) Day-release programmes. *Update* **15**, 1035–8.

Appendix F People and institutions suitable for trainees to visit

Family Practitioner Committee
G.P. Hospital
Industrial retraining unit
School for physically handicapped
School for emotionally disturbed
Centre for the education of deaf children
Old Peoples' Home
Hospice for the dying
Psychiatric day hospital
Drug Addiction Unit
Youth Counselling Service
Social work unit/Social Services
Regional Medical Officer
Samaritans
Youth Club
Red Cross/St John's
Citizens' Advice Bureau
Cruse Club (for widows)
Disabled Living Foundation (London)
Industrial Health and Safety Centre (London)
Regional employment medical officer
District medical officer
Community physicians
Hospital for mentally subnormal
Rehabilitation centre
Spastics centre
Cheshire Home
Halfway hostels
Sheltered workshop
Prison
Coalmine
Factory
Therapeutic community
Child Guidance Clinic
Probation Office
Magistrates Court
Coroner
Alcoholics Anonymous
Gamblers Anonymous
Rotary Club
Chemist
Public Health Department
Family Planning Association
Wolfson Institute (London)
Undertaker

Appendix G Basic reading list

There is an excellent and comprehensive booklist available from the British Postgraduate Medical Federation. The following selections are suggested as the beginnings of a reading programme, the further stages of which should be discussed and planned with your trainer.

The concept of training and its aims

The Future General Practitioner—Working Party, R.C.G.P. London, R.C.G.P. 1972. This book is a definitive guide to the purposes of vocational training. It is not the easiest of books to read and may be best taken a little at a time. Originally intended for teachers of general practice, parts of it are valuable reading for the trainee.

The setting of general practice

Manual of Primary Health Care by Peter Prichard (1978) Oxford University Press, Oxford. A wide ranging book that establishes the scenery and climate of modern general practice together with a lot of basic information on the 'nuts and bolts'.

An Introduction to Primary Medical Care by David C. Morrell (1981) London, Churchill Livingstone. A useful guide to who does what for the early days of a traineeship. This should be read early in the course.

An Introduction to Family Medicine by Ian R. McWhinney (1981) Oxford, Oxford University Press. This book is the distillation of years of research and experience by an eminent British GP who has become an even more eminent Canadian Professor of Family Medicine. Well worth reading not only for the approaches demonstrated but because it opens the door to work being done in primary care outside the UK.

The work of general practice

Trends in General Practice edited by John Fry (1979) London, RCGP. An analytical approach to the workload of the GP. An invaluable source of facts. A book for dipping into rather than reading.

The doctor and the patient

The Doctor, His Patient and the Illness by Michael Balint (1968) London, Pitman Medical. The original 'Bible' of modern general practice and, as such, an essential item of reading. Some of the ideas have become so well accepted as to be redundant in a teaching sense but as a landmark this book must be read.

The Doctor/Patient Relationship by Kevin Browne and Paul Freeling (1976) London, Churchill Livingstone. This is the accepted basic textbook on this important subject (Yes, we are biased) and should be read during the early part of the trainee year.

Clinical medicine in general practice

Towards Earlier Diagnosis by Keith Hodgkin (1978) London, Churchill Livingstone. A useful guide to the clinical method and problems of the GP. This book eases the transition from hospital to GP clinician.

Sociology

An Introduction to Medical Sociology, edited by David Tuckett (1976), London, Tavistock Publications Ltd. An easily-read guide that includes the basic terminology of the sciences and its application to general practice. Useful background material.

Sociology as Applied to Medicine, edited by Donald L. Patrick and Graham Scrambler (1982) Baillière's Concise Medical Textbooks. This book takes a slightly different approach to that of Tuckett and includes helpful information on ethnic groups.

Practice administration and finance

Running a Practice, by Robert Jones et al. (1978) London, Croom Helm. A book for the latter part of the year before the trainee starts to look for his own practice. A valuable 'Which' guide to practices. A compact but comprehensive guide to organization and management that fills in the details missing from some of the above.

Research

Research in General Practice, by John Howie (1979) London, Croom Helm. A guide to the possibilities of GP research well illustrated with actual examples.

Survey Methods in Community Medicine, by J. H. Abramson (1974) London, Churchill Livingstone.

And finally

Help! I can't cope

A Guide to General Practice—The Oxford G.P. Trainee Group (1979). Oxford, Blackwell Scientific Publications. A practical guide to the administrative and clinical problems that may be met during the trainee year. Written by recent trainees. Keep it in the car!

References

Abramson J. H. (1974) *Survey Methods in Community Medicine.* London, Churchill Livingstone.

Balint M. (1957) *The Doctor, his Patient and the Illness.* London, Pitman Medical.

Bugden J. A. (1977) *The Health Visitor.* Personal communication.

Byrne P. S. and Long B. L. (1976) *Doctors talking to Patients.* London, HMSO.

Crombie D. L. and Pinsent R. J. F. H. (1976) The nature of information used in making clinical decisions in general practice. *J. R. Coll. Gen. Pract.* **26**, 502–6.

Donabedian A. (1976) Evaluating the quality of medical care. *Millbank Memorial Fund Quarterly* Part 2; **49**, 166 *et seq.*

Durkin C. J. and Edwards A. (1975) Referral letters from general practitioners. *J. R. Coll. Gen. Pract.* **25**, 532–6.

General Medical Council (1980) *Recommendations as to Basic Medical Education.*

Graham J. M. and Supree D. A. (1979) Improving drug compliance in general practice. *J. R. Coll. Gen. Pract.* **29**, 399–404.

Green R. H. (1973) General practitioners and open-access pathology services. *J. R. Coll. Gen. Pract.* **23**, 316–25.

Green R. H. (1976) An experimental service for pathology specimens. *J. R. Coll. Gen. Pract.* **26**, 185–91.

Hasler J. C. (1982) *Clinical Experience of Trainees in General Practice.* Unpublished MD Thesis.

Heron J. (1975) *Six Categories of Intervention Analysis.* Guildford, University of Surrey.

Hodgkin K. (1979) Diagnosis vocabulary for primary care. *J. Fam. Pract.* **8**, 129–44.

Howie J. G. R. (1974) Clinical judgement and antibiotic use in general practice. *Br. Med. J.* **2**, 1061–4.

Leavell H. R. and Clark E. G. (1965) *Preventive Medicine for the Doctor in his Community.* New York, McGraw-Hill.

Leeuwenhorst Working Party (1974) The General Practitioner in Europe. *J. R. Coll. Gen. Pract.* **27**, 117.

Ley P. (1979) Memory for medical information. *Br. J. Soc. Clin. Psychol.* **18**, 245–55.

Marinker M. L. (1976–81) In: Cormack J., Marinker M. L. and Morrell D. C. (ed.) *Health and Unhealth in Practice: A Handbook of Primary Medical Care.* London, Kluwer-Harrap Handbooks.

Marsh G. N. (1982) Are follow-up consultations at medical outpatients futile? *Br. Med. J.* **1**, 1176–7.

Morrell D. C., Gaze H. G. and Robinson N. A. (1971) Symptoms in general practice. *J. R. Coll. Gen. Pract.* **21**, 52–3.

Office of Health Economics (1975) *Compendium of Health Statistics*, p. 37.

Parish P. A. (1971) The prescribing of psychotropic drugs in general practice. *J. R. Coll. Gen. Pract.* **21**, Suppl. 4.

Parish P. A., Williams W. M. and Elmer P. C. (1973) The medical use of psychotropic drugs. *J. R. Coll. Gen. Pract.* **21**, Suppl. 4.

Patterson R. H., Fraser R. C. and Peacock E. (1974) Diagnostic procedures and the general practitioner. *J. R. Coll. Gen. Pract.* **24**, 237–41.

Pendleton D. A., Schofield T. P. C. and Tate P. H. L. (1982) *The Consultation: an Approach to Learning and Teaching.* Oxford, Oxford University Press.

Reedy B. L. E. C., Metcalfe A. U., de Roumanine M. et al. (1980a) The social and occupational characteristics of attached and employed nurses in general practice. *J. R. Coll. Gen. Pract.* **30**, 473–82.

Reedy B. L. E. C., Metcalfe A. U., de Roumaine M. et al. (1980b). A comparison of the activities and opinions of attached and employed nurses in general practice. *J. R. Coll. Gen. Pract.* **30**, 483–9.

Royal College of General Practitioners (1972) *The Future General Practitioner—Learning and Teaching*. London, British Medical Journal.

Royal College of General Practitioners Census and Surveys and The Department of Health and Social Security (1974) *Morbidity Statistics from General Practice. Second National Morbidity Study. 1970–71*. London, HMSO.

Royal College of General Practitioners (1977) *Better Clinical Standards. Report of a Working Party of the Board of Census to the Council of the Royal College of General Practitioners*. London, privately circulated.

Royal College of General Practitioners (1979) *Trends in General Practice, 1979*. 2nd ed. London, British Medical Association.

Royal College of General Practitioners (1981) *Anticipatory Care. Reports from General Practice, 18*. February.

Scott J. Bodley (1965) The Bedside Manner. *Trans. Med. Soc. Lond.* **193**, 1–12.

Smith G. L. (1979) An evaluation of direct access radiology in general practice. *J. R. Coll. Gen. Pract.* **29**, 539–45.

Stott N. C. H. (1979) Management and outcome of winter upper respiratory tract infections in children aged 0–9 years. *Br. Med. J.* **1**, 29–31.

Stott N. C. H. and Davis R. H. (1979) The exceptional potential of each primary care consultation. *J. R. Coll. Gen. Pract.* **29**, 201–5.

Szasz T. and Hollender M. (1956) A contribution to the philosophy of medicine: the basic models of the doctor-patient relationship. *Arch. Int. Med.* **97**, 585.

Tait I. (1974). Person-centred perspectives in medicine. *J. R. Coll. Gen. Pract.* **24**, 151–60.

Taylor R. J. (1977) General practice prescribing. *J. R. Coll. Gen. Pract.* **27**, 79–82.

Taylor R. J. (1978) Prescribing costs and patterns of prescribing in general practice. *J. R. Coll. Gen. Pract.* **28**, 531–5.

Thomson G. H. (1978) Tolerating uncertainty in family medicine. *J. R. Coll. Gen. Pract.* **28**, 343–6.

Tuckett D. (1976) *An Introduction to Medical Sociology*. London, Tavistock Publications.

Varnam M. A. (1981) Psychotropic prescribing. What am I doing? *J. R. Coll. Gen. Pract.* **31**, 480–3.

Wallace B. S., Millward D., Parsons A. S. et al. (1973) Unrestricted access by general practitioners to a department of diagnostic radiology. *J. R. Coll. Gen. Pract.* **23**, 337–43.

Woodcock J. (1970) In: Balint M., Hunt J., Joyce D. et al (ed.) *Differences in the Doctor's Prescribing Habits in Treatment or Diagnosis: a Study of Repeat Prescriptions in General Practice*. London, Tavistock Publications.

INDEX